T0362281

Modern Approaches to Facial and Athletic Injuries

Editors

J. DAVID KRIET

CLINTON D. HUMPHREY

FACIAL PLASTIC SURGERY CLINICS OF NORTH AMERICA

www.facialplastic.theclinics.com

Consulting Editor
J. REGAN THOMAS

February 2022 • Volume 30 • Number 1

ELSEVIER

1600 John F. Kennedy Boulevard • Suite 1800 • Philadelphia, Pennsylvania, 19103-2899

http://www.theclinics.com

FACIAL PLASTIC SURGERY CLINICS OF NORTH AMERICA Volume 30, Number 1
February 2022 ISSN 1064-7406, ISBN-13: 978-0-323-89714-3

Editor: Stacy Eastman
Developmental Editor: Ann Gielou M. Posedio

Facial Plastic Surgery Clinics of North America (ISSN 1064-7406) is published quarterly by Elsevier Inc., 360 Park Avenue South, New York, NY 10010-1710. Months of issue are February, May, August, and November. Business and Editorial Offices: 1600 John F. Kennedy Blvd., Suite 1800, Philadelphia, PA 19103-2899. Periodicals postage paid at New York, NY, and additional mailing offices. Subscription prices are $420.00 per year (US individuals), $922.00 per year (US institutions), $468.00 per year (Canadian individuals), $950.00 per year (Canadian institutions), $557.00 per year (foreign individuals), $950.00 per year (foreign institutions), $100.00 per year (US students), $100.00 per year (Canadian students), and $255.00 per year (foreign students). Foreign air speed delivery is included in all *Clinics* subscription prices. All prices are subject to change without notice. POSTMASTER: Send address changes to *Facial Plastic Surgery Clinics*, Elsevier Health Sciences Division, Subscription Customer Service, 3251 Riverport Lane, Maryland Heights, MO 63043. **Customer service: 1-800-654-2452 (US and Canada); 1-314-447-8871 (outside US and Canada); Fax: 314-447-8029; E-mail: journalscustomerservice-usa@elsevier.com (for print support); journalsonlinesupport-usa@elsevier.com (for online support).**

Reprints. For copies of 100 or more of articles in this publication, please contact the Commercial Reprints Department, Elsevier Inc., 360 Park Avenue South, New York, NY 10010-1710. Tel.: 212-633-3874; Fax: 212-633-3820; E-mail: reprints@elsevier.com.

Facial Plastic Surgery Clinics of North America is covered in *MEDLINE/PubMed* (*Index Medicus*).

Contributors

CONSULTING EDITOR

J. REGAN THOMAS, MD
Professor, Facial Plastic and Reconstructive
Surgery, Department of Otolaryngology–Head
and Neck Surgery, Northwestern University
Feinberg School of Medicine, Chicago, Illinois

EDITORS

J. DAVID KRIET, MD, FACS
WS and EC Jones Endowed Professor,
Director, Division of Facial Plastic Surgery,
Department of Otolaryngology, University of
Kansas Health System, Kansas City, Kansas

CLINTON D. HUMPHREY, MD, FACS
Associate Professor, Division of Facial Plastic
Surgery, Department of Otolaryngology,
University of Kansas Health System, Kansas
City, Kansas

AUTHORS

BENJAMIN T. BARBETTA, DMD, MD
Program Director, Henry Ford Oral and
Maxillofacial Surgery, Senior Staff Surgeon,
Henry Ford Health System, Detroit, Michigan

SYDNEY C. BUTTS, MD, FACS
Associate Professor and Chief, Facial Plastic
and Reconstructive Surgery, Division of Facial
Plastic and Reconstructive Surgery,
Department of Otolaryngology, SUNY
Downstate Health Sciences University, Kings
County Hospital Center, Brooklyn, New York

JUNGSUK CHO, DMD, MD
Assistant Professor of Oral and Maxillofacial
Surgery, Temple University School of Dentistry,
Pittsburgh, Pennsylvania

LARRY L. CUNNINGHAM, Jr, DDS, MD
Professor and Chair, Oral and Maxillofacial
Surgery, University of Pittsburgh School of
Dental Medicine, Pittsburgh, Pennsylvania

RAJ D. DEDHIA, MD
Department of Otolaryngology–Head and Neck
Surgery, University of Tennessee, Memphis,
Tennessee

JAMES ENG, MD
Resident Physician, Bobby R. Alford
Department of Otolaryngology–Head and Neck
Surgery, Baylor College of Medicine, Houston,
Texas

JOHN FLYNN, MD
Department of Otolaryngology–Head and Neck
Surgery, University of Kansas School of
Medicine, The University of Kansas Medical
Center, Kansas City, Kansas

RAHUL D. GULATI, MD
Resident, Department of Otolaryngology,
SUNY Downstate Health Sciences University,
Brooklyn, New York

STEVEN G. HOSHAL, MD
Department of Otolaryngology –Head and
Neck Surgery, University of California, Davis,
Sacramento, California

CHRISTINE M. JONES, MD
Assistant Professor, Division of Plastic and
Reconstructive Surgery, Lewis Katz School of
Medicine at Temple University, Philadelphia,
Pennsylvania

LAMONT R. JONES, MD, MBA, FACS
Executive Vice Chair, Department of Otolaryngology–Head and Neck Surgery, Facial Plastic and Reconstructive Surgery, Co-Director, Cleft and Craniofacial Clinic, Medical Director, Ambulatory Surgery, Henry Ford Health System, Otolaryngology Service Chief, Henry Ford West Bloomfield Hospital, Clinical Associate Professor, Wayne State University School of Medicine, Henry Ford Health System, Detroit, Michigan

ANDREW S. KAO, MS
Medical Student, Wayne State University School of Medicine, Detroit, Michigan

VINCENT H. KEY, MD
Associate Professor, Orthopaedic Surgery/Sports Medicine, University of Kansas Health System, Kansas City, Kansas

SARAH MAZHER KIDWAI, MD
Otolaryngologist/Facial Plastic Surgeon, Northwell Long Island Jewish Medical Center, Assistant Professor, Donald and Barbara Zucker School of Medicine at Hofstra/Northwell, New Hyde Park, New York

KYLE KIMURA, MD
Resident Physician, Department of Otolaryngology–Head and Neck Surgery, Vanderbilt University Medical Center, Nashville, Tennessee

KELLY C. LANDEEN, MD
Resident Physician, Department of Otolaryngology–Head and Neck Surgery, Vanderbilt University Medical Center, Nashville, Tennessee

KATHERINE A. LARRABEE, MD
House Office, Henry Ford Health System, Detroit, Michigan

G. NINA LU, MD
Assistant Professor, Division of Facial Plastic and Reconstructive Surgery, Department of Otolaryngology–Head and Neck Surgery, University of Washington, Harborview Medical Center, Seattle, Washington

SEAN MOONEY, MD
Resident, Department of Otolaryngology, SUNY Downstate Health Sciences University, Brooklyn, New York

ANDREW H. MURR, MD, FACS
Professor and Chairman, Department of Otolaryngology–Head and Neck Surgery, University of California, San Francisco, School of Medicine, Attending Staff, Zuckerberg San Francisco General Hospital, San Francisco, California

JOSEPH B. NOLAND, MD
Assistant Professor, Family Medicine, University of Kansas Health System, Kansas City, Kansas

ALEX SACHS, DMD
Resident in Oral and Maxillofacial Surgery, University of Pittsburgh School of Dental Medicine, Pittsburgh, Pennsylvania

CECELIA E. SCHMALBACH, MD, MSc, FRCS
David Myers, MD Professor and Chair, Department of Otolaryngology–Head and Neck Surgery, Lewis Katz School of Medicine at Temple University, Philadelphia, Pennsylvania

DOUGLAS M. SIDLE, MD, FACS
Assistant Professor, Northwestern Department of Head and Neck Surgery, Division of Facial Plastic and Reconstructive Surgery, Chicago, Illinois

SUNTHOSH SIVAM, MD
Assistant Professor, Division of Facial Plastic and Reconstructive Surgery, Bobby R. Alford Department of Otolaryngology–Head and Neck Surgery, Baylor College of Medicine, Houston, Texas

GAELEN STANFORD-MOORE, MD
Resident, Department of Otolaryngology–Head and Neck Surgery, University of California, San Francisco, School of Medicine, San Francisco, California

SCOTT J. STEPHAN, MD
Chief, Division of Facial Plastic and Reconstructive Surgery, Department of Otolaryngology–Head and Neck Surgery, Vanderbilt University Medical Center, Nashville, Tennessee

E. BRADLEY STRONG, MD
Professor, Department of Otolaryngology–Head and Neck Surgery, University of California, Davis, Sacramento, California

STEVE YUSUPOV, DDS, MD, FACS
Director, Maxillofacial Oncology, Staten Island
University Hospital, Northwell Health,
Brooklyn, New York

ZACHARY A. ZIMMERMAN, MD
Facial Plastic and Reconstructive Surgery
Fellow, Northwestern Department of Head and
Neck Surgery, Division of Facial Plastic and
Reconstructive Surgery, Chicago, Illinois

Contents

supports a paradigm shift from open surgical management to a more conservative treatment algorithm emphasizing observation and minimally invasive endoscopic techniques. Long-term follow-up for complex frontal sinus injuries is critical

Mandibular Condylar Fractures   85

Sean Mooney, Rahul D. Gulati, Steve Yusupov, and Sydney C. Butts

Mandibular condyle fractures can result in short-term and long-term morbidity. As a weak area of the mandible, the condyle is vulnerable to injury by a direct impact or an indirect force. Current treatment recommendations aim to better match the severity of the fracture with the choice of closed or open approach. Long-term follow-up of patients provides the best opportunity to monitor the degree of functional restoration after treatment. There is a growing consensus regarding the use of standardized fracture classification methods and outcomes measures that will allow better assessment of treatment results and strengthen the quality of outcomes research.

Mandibular Body Fractures   99

Sarah Mazher Kidwai and G. Nina Lu

Fractures of the mandibular body most commonly occur after interpersonal violence or motorized vehicle accident but can occur in athletes. Mandibular body fractures are often associated with additional mandibular fractures. The treatment goal is to achieve preinjury occlusion and facial appearance, and this can be done via a closed reduction and maxillomandibular fixation or open reduction and fixation with or without maxillomandibular fixation. The authors present 3 cases in this article.

Mandibular Angle Fractures   109

Gaelen Stanford-Moore and Andrew H. Murr

Angle fractures are the most common among the mandibular fractures. History and physical examination are crucial in guiding time course and specifics of manage- ment. Computed tomography (CT) has become the gold standard for diagnosis of mandible fractures, offering advantages for both surgical planning and assessing dental involvement. Currently the use of a single monocortical plate with the Champy technique for osteosynthesis is used preferentially for noncomminuted fractures of the mandibular angle. Other load-sharing options for plating include strut plates, malleable plates, and geometric or 3D plates. Load-bearing options remain viable for comminuted fractures or other complex circumstances.

Dental Trauma and Alveolar Fractures   117

Jungsuk Cho, Alex Sachs, and Larry L. Cunningham Jr

A dentoalveolar fracture requires thorough clinical and radiographic examination for an accurate diagnosis to guide appropriate treatment. Dentoalveolar fractures can be classified into the following 4 groups: (1) crown/root fractures, (2) luxation/ displacement of teeth, (3) avulsion, and (4) alveolar fractures. Treatment can be divided into nonrigid fixation (splinting with wires and composite) and/or rigid fixation (Erich arch bars, Risdon cable wires) depending on the extent of dentoalveolar frac- tures. Special considerations must be made for primary teeth and mixed dentition to avoid injuring tooth buds and arising permanent dentition.

FACIAL PLASTIC SURGERY CLINICS OF NORTH AMERICA

FORTHCOMING ISSUES

RECENT ISSUES

SERIES OF RELATED INTEREST

Clinics in Plastic Surgery
https://www.plasticsurgery.theclinics.com
Otolaryngologic Clinics
https://www.oto.theclinics.com
Dermatologic Clinics
https://www.derm.theclinics.com

THE CLINICS ARE AVAILABLE ONLINE!
Access your subscription at:
www.theclinics.com

Foreword
Modern Approaches to Facial and Athletic Injuries

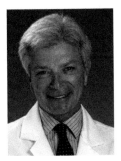

J. Regan Thomas, MD
Consulting Editor

Facial trauma and injuries are frequent occurrences related to all types of athletic and sports activities. Both adults and children sustain facial injuries through athletic activities relatively frequently and often require treatment by facial plastic and reconstructive surgeons as well as general otolaryngologists, oral and maxillofacial surgeons, and plastic surgeons. When significant facial injuries are sustained by our patients, they often require evaluation and possible treatment for other injuries, such as concussion, ocular injuries, and dental areas of concern. Appropriate evaluation and potential treatment by a team of specialists are frequently a consideration that is often led by the facial plastic and reconstructive surgeon who has had the initial contact with the individual sustaining facial trauma from athletic activities.

Facial soft tissue injuries, including lacerations, hematoma, and even tissue avulsion, may be the initial or primary concern from facial athletic trauma. The responsible facial plastic surgeon should have the skills and knowledge base to effectively treat these injuries that frequently are sustained from athletic activity trauma. Facial fractures and facial bone anatomy injuries are very frequent and require appropriate evaluation, diagnosis, and treatment. Indeed, it is not unusual for the patient to require treatment for both soft tissue and facial bone injuries. Accordingly, the facial plastic surgeon should have the expertise and insight to both treat these injuries and coordinate other requirements of care for the facially injured athlete.

As guest editors for this issue's topics, Dr Kriet and Dr Humphrey have assembled an expert group of experienced and knowledgeable contributing authors to cover this wide array, but related topics. Although these facial injuries and their required care and treatment can happen from a variety of causes, athletic activities are frequently the cause. This issue's authors are all experienced and recognized experts in their areas of discussion.

This issue of *Facial Plastic Surgery Clinics of North America* as organized by Dr Kriet and Dr Humphrey provides a valuable and pragmatic reference for those physicians providing care in this very common area of athletic facial trauma. I am quite pleased to provide this well-organized and expert review of this growing area of facial surgical practice to our readership.

J. Regan Thomas, MD
Facial Plastic and Reconstructive Surgery
Department of Otolaryngology–
Head and Neck Surgery
Northwestern University School of Medicine
60 East Delaware Place
Chicago, IL 60611, USA

E-mail address:
regan.thomas@nm.org

Facial Plast Surg Clin N Am 30 (2022) xi
https://doi.org/10.1016/j.fsc.2021.09.002
1064-7406/22/© 2021 Published by Elsevier Inc.

facialplastic.theclinics.com

Preface
Managing Craniomaxillofacial Injuries in Athletes

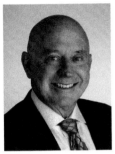

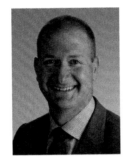

J. David Kriet, MD, FACS   Clinton D. Humphrey, MD, FACS
Editors

Competitive athletics remain immensely popular in our society among both youth and adults. Head and facial injuries are common during athletic activities, and the expertise of the facial trauma surgeon is frequently sought to treat these injuries. Facial injuries may account for up to 29% of athletic injuries, and 11% to 42% of all facial fractures are acquired during athletic activities. Soft tissue injuries and nasal bone fractures are most common. However, other injuries, such as zygomaticomaxillary, orbital, mandible, midface, and frontal sinus fractures, frequently occur.

In this issue of *Facial Plastic Surgery Clinics of North America*, we sought to provide practicing surgeons with information about the current best evidence-based practices for making challenging decisions about airway management, anesthesia, and ideal timing for treatment of maxillofacial injuries in athletes. Another challenge is the best approach to managing the teeth in isolated or concurrent dental injuries. Oral and maxillofacial surgeons provide guidance for treating these patients in an article on dental fractures and alveolar trauma. Utilizing new technology, such as

Facial Plast Surg Clin N Am 30 (2022) xiii–xiv
https://doi.org/10.1016/j.fsc.2021.09.001
1064-7406/22/© 2021 Published by Elsevier Inc.

intraoperative CT and virtual surgical planning, that reduces operative time and improves patient outcomes is discussed in the article on orbital fractures.

Unique to maxillofacial injuries, especially in the most competitive athletes, are questions about when "return to play" is appropriate. The facial trauma surgeon may not be the final authority on such questions particularly when there is a known concussion. Nonetheless, the surgeon's opinion will still often be sought by athletes, trainers, coaches, and parents. Familiarity with the appropriate testing and protocols used in making these decisions is useful. An orthopedic surgeon and sports medicine physician provide their insights to this process in their article on concussion in the athlete and return-to-play guidelines.

Athletes with maxillofacial injuries have particular needs and concerns. We hope that this issue of *Facial Plastic Surgery Clinics of North America* will help the facial trauma surgeon fully develop the specific skill set required for comprehensive care of these patients.

J. David Kriet, MD, FACS
Division of Facial Plastic Surgery
Department of Otolaryngology
University of Kansas Health System
3901 Rainbow Boulevard
MS 3010
Kansas City, KS 66160, USA

Clinton D. Humphrey, MD, FACS
Division of Facial Plastic Surgery
Department of Otolaryngology
University of Kansas Health System
3901 Rainbow Boulevard
MS 3010
Kansas City, KS 66160, USA

E-mail addresses:
dkriet@kumc.edu (J.D. Kriet)
chumphrey@kumc.edu (C.D. Humphrey)
www.kufacialplasticsurgery.com

General Overview of the Facial Trauma Evaluation

James Eng, MD, Sunthosh Sivam, MD*

KEYWORDS

- Maxillofacial trauma • Facial fractures • Primary survey • Airway emergency • Initial management

KEY POINTS

- Following Advanced Trauma Life Support (ATLS) guidelines is paramount in the management of patients with facial trauma.
- Establishing and maintaining a safe airway precedes all other interventions. Facial trauma specifically can create tenuous airways requiring multiple modalities or techniques for the management.
- A thorough head and neck examination, including a neurologic and ophthalmologic examination, can provide insight into underlying maxillofacial fractures.
- Nasal injuries are the most common facial injuries across all sports. Epistaxis management includes pressure, packing, and ultimately ligation or embolization.
- Computed tomography is the gold standard for the radiographic evaluation of maxillofacial trauma.

INTRODUCTION

In the United States (US), each year, more than 400,000 emergency room visits are related to facial injuries, up to 30% of which may be sports-related. The National Youth Sports Foundation for the Prevention of Athletics Injuries in the US estimates that athletes have a 10% chance of sustaining maxillofacial injury during each sports season.[1,2] These injuries are complex, and although rarely life-threatening, can affect the functionality or cosmesis of the face.

Previous studies have shown that 11% to 40% of all sports-related injuries involve the face. These injuries may be related to falls, interplayer contacts, and impacts from sporting equipment. In the US, sports-specific patterns of injury in adults are not well established; among the pediatric population, more than 43% of facial trauma is attributed to baseball or softball. Throughout the world, cultural and socioeconomic differences contribute to the variability of trends in sports popularity and resultant sports-related injuries. As such, most injuries occur from soccer in Italy and France, basketball in Japan, soccer in South Korea, ice hockey in Finland, and skiing in Austria and Switzerland.[2–4]

Soft tissue injuries, as well as facial bone fractures, occur frequently in athletes with the nasal bone, mandible, and zygoma being the most common subsites. Nasal bone fractures account for up to 50% of all sports-related fractures, whereas zygomaticomaxillary complex (ZMC) and mandibular fractures each account for another 10%.[5] The type of sport can also influence maxillofacial fracture patterns which was illustrated in a German study of 3596 patients showing that ball sport accidents lead to significantly more midface fractures than mandibular fractures.[3]

Prompt evaluation by a facial plastic surgeon can allow for the early recognition of maxillofacial trauma that may require emergent intervention. Early surgical intervention, when indicated, has been demonstrated to improve esthetic and functional outcomes.[6] The ultimate goal of the facial trauma surgeon is the restoration of the face and its functions to the preinjury state.

Division of Facial Plastic & Reconstructive Surgery, Bobby R. Alford Department of Otolaryngology-Head and Neck Surgery, Baylor College of Medicine, 1977 Butler Boulevard, Suite E5.200, Houston, TX 77030, USA
* Corresponding author.
E-mail address: sunthosh.sivam@bcm.edu

Facial Plast Surg Clin N Am 30 (2022) 1–9
https://doi.org/10.1016/j.fsc.2021.08.001
1064-7406/22/© 2021 Elsevier Inc. All rights reserved.

PRIMARY SURVEY

Approximately 25% to 30% of trauma-related deaths can be prevented by using a systematic approach to evaluating the patient.[7] The goal of the initial trauma assessment is to recognize life-threatening injuries and establish an organized treatment plan to aggressively manage urgent issues. When considering patients with trauma as a whole, injuries are missed in up to 65% of patients.[8] For this reason, following the stabilization of the patient, the trauma team should perform serial examination to avoid missing injuries.[6]

On arrival, a history of the patient's mechanism of injury, vital signs, and interventions provided in the field should be clearly communicated from the emergency medical services (EMS) team to the receiving hospital care team. The mechanism of injury can provide clues into different patterns of facial fractures and insight into other underlying injuries that may not be immediately recognized. For example, high-velocity motor vehicle collisions more commonly cause complex and multifocal fractures than falls, fights, or sports-related injuries.[4,9,10]

Following the transfer of the patient to the trauma bay bed, the usual sequence of events includes the primary survey, the stabilization of the patient, the secondary survey, and the establishment of a definitive care plan. The most common system to describe a patient's status is the Glasgow Coma Scale (GCS). Patients with a GCS score between 3 and 8 require urgent management, generally including endotracheal intubation. Ensuring airway protection may still be indicated in patients with GCS score greater than 8 in the case of maxillofacial trauma causing airway compromise.[7]

The primary survey is based on the "ABCDEs" of trauma as described by the American College of Surgeons Advanced Trauma Life Support: Airway, Breathing, Circulation, Disability, and Exposure.[1,6,7] We will focus our discussion on the first 3 and how they pertain to patients with maxillofacial trauma.

"A" FOR AIRWAY ASSESSMENT AND MANAGEMENT
Assessing the Airway

Determining airway patency is of utmost importance, especially in patients with head and neck injuries or maxillofacial trauma. Poor systemic oxygen delivery can lead to loss of consciousness, end-organ failure, and ultimately death. An easy way to quickly determine airway adequacy is by assessing a patient's ability to respond to questions.[11,12] A patient that is lying flat and able to speak with normal vocal projection and without too frequent of breaks in speech to catch their breath likely has a patent airway.

The thyroid cartilage should be assessed for midline positioning and irregularities that suggest a fracture. Crepitus felt in the neck or air bubbles emerging from a neck wound may result from a tracheal injury. Maxillofacial trauma can contribute to airway obstruction from bleeding, posterior mobility of the maxilla to the nasopharynx, prolapse of the tongue to the posterior oropharynx in mandibular fractures, or displaced dentition, and other foreign bodies.[13] Not surprisingly, it has been previously shown that complex fractures are more commonly associated with airway compromise and the need for tracheostomy.[10] Other potential causes of airway obstruction include emesis, lingual edema, and traumatic brain injury.

Signs and symptoms of airway obstruction include

- Agitation or use of accessory respiratory muscles
- A need to preferentially sit upright
- Rapid shallow breaths
- Hypoxia demonstrated on pulse oximetry
- Cyanosis suggesting hypercarbia
- Stridor
- Deviated laryngotracheal framework
- Options for securing the airway are discussed below and summarized in **Fig. 1**

Nonsurgical Airway Management

Initially, patients are provided with supplemental oxygen via mask or nasal cannula. Placement of a nasopharyngeal (NPA) or oropharyngeal (OPA) airway is a quick adjunct to bypass an enlarged tongue. If more airway support is required, the bag valve mask is an essential tool because it provides positive pressure ventilation and can even act as a definitive airway if used correctly.

Escalation of airway management then moves to intubation. A greater number of facial fractures and more complex fracture patterns both confer an increased risk of cervical spine injury.[14] If a cervical collar must be removed to establish a definitive airway, another team member should manually stabilize the head and neck. The jaw thrust and chin lift are 2 maneuvers that can assist in safely opening the oral airway without compromising the spine.[15]

In brief, orotracheal intubation typically involves direct or video laryngoscopy followed by the placement of an endotracheal tube (ETT). Appropriate positioning of the tube can be confirmed

Options for Securing the Airway

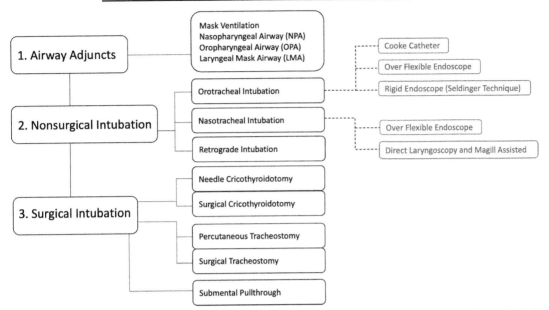

Fig. 1. Multiple tools and methods exist for establishing a safe and secure airway in patients with maxillofacial trauma. The decision on which technique to use depends on individual patient circumstances, available resources, existing injuries, other contraindications for certain techniques, and practitioner comfort and preference.

by the visualization of the tube passing through the vocal folds, end-tidal carbon dioxide using capnography, and bilateral auscultation for even respiratory sounds. Once the positioning is confirmed, the tube should be properly secured.

When standard orotracheal intubation is difficult, other options exist before obtaining a surgical airway. A small diameter elastic bougie can pass through the glottis more easily. An ETT is then passed over the bougie into position. Rescue airway devices including the laryngeal mask airway (LMA) or fiberoptic intubation are alternatives. Nasotracheal intubation using a fiberoptic scope is a good option for patients with a potentially difficult airway (**Fig. 2**) who must maintain spontaneous ventilation. This method is occasionally contraindicated in the case of midface and skull-base trauma because of the risk of brain injury or cerebrospinal fluid leak.

Retrograde intubation may be considered when a flexible scope is not available or bleeding makes scope visualization difficult. A thin guide wire is passed through the cricothyroid membrane and aimed cephalad, passing through the glottis into the oral cavity. A flexible ETT can then be passed over the guide until its tip is engaged at the laryngeal inlet. While applying axial pressure over the ETT tip to hold it in place, the guide is removed and the ETT is then advanced distally into the trachea.[16]

The Surgical Airway

In certain cases, intubation may not be possible and obtaining a surgical airway may be necessary. One of the fastest means of obtaining an airway is with a cricothyroidotomy. This involves an incision through the cricothyroid membrane, followed by the dilation of the tract to accommodate a small ETT.[17] A needle cricothyroidotomy is also an option; however, this is only a temporizing measure. A needle cricothyroidotomy can facilitate translaryngeal jet ventilation for approximately 30 minutes, with hypercarbia noted beyond that time.[13]

Tracheostomy is preferentially performed in children to avoid injury to the cricoid cartilage during a cricothyroidotomy. For practitioners with advanced training in airway management, expeditious awake tracheostomy may be an option even in an unstable patient.

The surgical plan itself can dictate subsequent airway management after securing the airway at the time of presentation. For mandibulomaxillary fixation (MMF), nasotracheal intubation or tracheostomy is often indicated; however, orotracheal tube may be routed behind the dentition still allowing for MMF. Alternatively, a submental pullthrough involving tunneling an oral ETT through the floor of the mouth and submental soft tissues may also be a viable option.[18] Lastly, as part of a multidisciplinary trauma team, it is prudent to

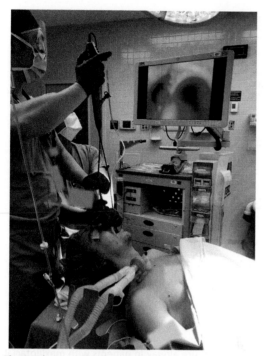

Fig. 2. Photograph of a patient with complex mandibular fractures undergoing nasotracheal intubation by the anesthesia and otolaryngology services using an ETT passed over a flexible fiberoptic scope. The scope allows for the visualization of distal airway structures, with the carina seen on the monitor, and confirmation of ETT placement. (*Courtesy of* Daniel Vinh, MD, Houston.)

consider tracheostomy for patients with polytrauma who may require prolonged intubation.

"B" FOR BREATHING

Once the airway has been secured, the patient should be assessed for adequate gas exchange to prevent hypoxemia and hypercarbia. Head injuries may affect respiratory drive, whereas spinal injuries above the levels of C3 to C5 may impact the phrenic nerves and subsequently the movements of the diaphragm. As a result, the neck and chest should be fully exposed to allow for adequate inspection and palpation with special attention to tracheal deviation, neck injuries, rib fractures, chest wall emphysema, and use of accessory muscles such as supraclavicular retractions.

Thoracic injuries including flail chest, hemothorax, and pneumothorax can also result in inadequate ventilation. If these injuries are suspected, a chest radiograph should be obtained promptly as needle decompression or chest tube placement may be necessary, especially in the case of a tension pneumothorax.

"C" FOR CIRCULATION

Hemorrhage accounts for 30% to 40% of preventable deaths in patients with trauma.[19] Resuscitation starts with establishing intravenous access with at least 2 large-bore intravenous catheters. Patients can initially receive crystalloid solutions; however, a blood transfusion may still be needed. Administration of blood products has the added benefit of repleting the circulatory system's oxygen-carrying capacity. Response to fluid resuscitation is assessed by monitoring the patient's vital signs, mental status, urinary output, and acid–base laboratories.[7]

The head and neck anatomy is well vascularized, and soft tissue injuries in this area can lead to significant bleeding. Up to 4.5% of patients with maxillofacial trauma experience life-threatening hemorrhage and subsequent hemorrhagic shock.[14] Scalp lacerations may be missed if the patient is hypovolemic, but when recognized can be quickly stabilized with Raney clips, staples, or sutures.[20] In the case of oral bleeding from mandibular fractures, bridle wires or arch bars can temporize the bleeding.

Epistaxis Management

In a review of 312 patients, Buchanan and colleagues found a 4% incidence of epistaxis across all facial fractures and an 11% incidence among midface fractures.[21] Nasal injuries are the most common facial injury across all sports, and both nasal bone fractures and isolated mucosal trauma can be associated with epistaxis.[3] Initial epistaxis management includes applying firm digital pressure over bilateral nasal ala and tilting the head forward to prevent OPA rundown, which can induce further anxiety, coughing, and emesis. Oxymetazoline (*Afrin*) is a topical decongestant that binds alpha-adrenergic receptors causing vasoconstriction and can be sprayed directly into the nares. Absorbable packing materials such as *Nasopore* and nonabsorbable packing materials such as *Merocel* can be used as adjuncts when digital pressure does not sufficiently control nasal bleeding.[22]

Formal packing such as *Rhino Rocket* can be used to control massive bleeding from posterior and anterior sources. Traditional packing for posterior epistaxis involves using a Foley catheter balloon to tamponade the bleed at the level of the choanae/nasopharynx. Occasionally, surgical exploration and ligation, or embolization by interventional radiology may be needed for offending vessels that are difficult to control with packing.[19]

SECONDARY SURVEY

Once the primary survey is completed and any life-threatening conditions are adequately managed, the secondary assessment is undertaken with a subjective and objective examination of the patient. A history of the incident and brief medical history should be obtained from the patient or from family members, friends, or witnesses. The objective portion of the assessment includes a thorough head and neck examination; determination of neurologic status; and examination of the chest, abdomen, and extremities.

Neurologic Examination

If the patient exhibits altered mentation, neurologic deficits, seizure activity, or brief loss of consciousness, a computed tomography (CT) scan of the head is required to assess intracranial injury.

The neurologic examination includes assessment for pupillary asymmetries, cranial nerve (CN) deficits, and any localizing signs. Deficits of CN I (olfactory) suggest injury to the cribriform plate. An ocular examination involves the assessment of vision mediated by CN II (optic), and movement of the orbit which is controlled by CN III (oculomotor), CN IV (trochlear), and CN VI (abducens). Discrepancies between bilateral facial sensations may suggest injuries to the branches of CN V (trigeminal).

Similarly, injury to CN VII (facial) would cause facial asymmetry. In an obtunded patient, a sternal rub may elicit a grimace revealing the dynamic facial function. As a general principle, suspected injuries to the branches of the facial nerve proximal to a vertical line drawn from the lateral canthus may benefit from surgical exploration, whereas injuries distal to this line are more likely to spontaneously recover function due to arborization.[1] The gag reflex can be used as a surrogate for CN IX (glossopharyngeal) and CN X (vagus) function. Checking strength with shrugging the shoulders and turning the head would elicit an injury to CN XI (spinal accessory), and asymmetry of tongue protrusion would suggest injury to CN XII (hypoglossal).

Orbital Examination

Examination of the orbit is crucial. Up to 40% of orbital blowout fractures may be associated with ocular injury, ranging from minor to major.[9] A preliminary ocular examination should evaluate pupil reactivity, globe position, visual acuity, range of extraocular movements for the evidence of entrapment, chemosis (swelling of the conjunctiva), and hyphema (blood within the anterior chamber). If any serious injury is suspected, the eyes should be protected adequately until a formal examination can be performed by an ophthalmologist, because any increased pressure onto an already compromised eye can lead to permanent vision changes.[14]

Examination for Facial Fractures and Lacerations

Starting at the apex of the scalp, the maxillofacial skeleton should be thoroughly and systematically inspected. Battle sign (ecchymoses over the mastoid), raccoon eyes (ecchymoses around the orbits), hemotympanum, and persistent clear or red-tinged rhinorrhea concerning cerebrospinal fluid leak are all signs of fractures of the skull base.

Asymmetries and swelling of portions of the face may provide clues to underlying facial fractures. These should be further assessed with palpation for step-offs or crepitus along the frontal bones; supraorbital, lateral, and inferior orbital rims; the nasal bones; malar prominences; zygomatic arches; the maxilla; and the mandible. **Figs. 3–5** depict an illustrative case.

The nose should be inspected with a nasal speculum and headlight to assess for a septal hematoma, which separates the mucoperichondrium from the underlying septal cartilage. A failure to identify and address a septal hematoma can compromise the vascular supply to the septal cartilage, causing consequences downstream such as a saddle nose deformity. In the same vein, auricular hematomas should be drained and bolstered with a pressure dressing to prevent necrosis of the underlying ear cartilage. These are particularly common in wrestling and mixed martial arts whereby shearing forces are applied to the external ear.[12]

Lacerations and avulsions should be thoroughly irrigated and closed within 4 to 6 hours if possible.[23] Occasionally, delayed primary closure is indicated for contaminated wounds, which should first be debrided, irrigated, and packed. In deep lacerations of the cheek, practitioners should probe the length of Stenson's duct, which carries saliva from the parotid gland to the oral cavity. Injuries to Stenson's duct can be identified by using a lacrimal probe, a small caliber catheter, or retrograde injection of methylene blue. These injuries can be managed with primary anastomosis, creation of an oral fistula for the diversion of salivary flow into the oral cavity, or medical suppression of saliva production. Primary anastomosis is the treatment of choice when possible, and can be performed over a lacrimal stent to prevent stenosis in the area of repair.[24] Adequate management of Stenson's duct injuries can prevent subsequent development of infection, sialocele, or fistula.[1]

Different physical examination findings can increase your suspicion for particular fracture patterns. For example, telecanthus, a more rounded

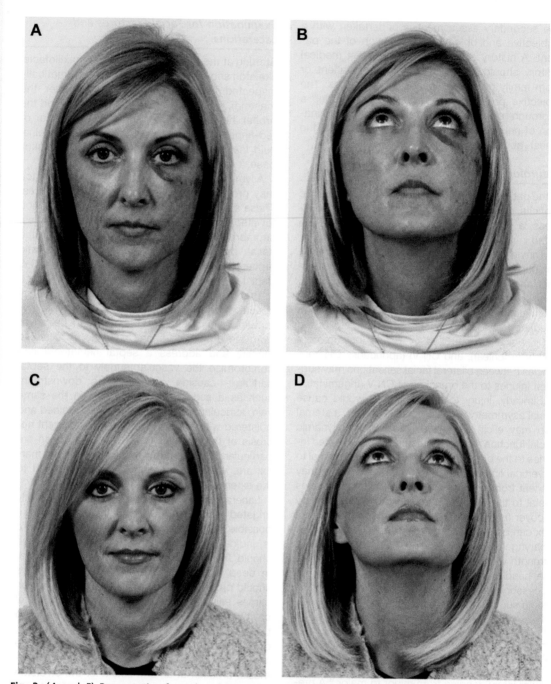

Fig. 3. (*A* and *B*) Preoperative frontal and base view photographs of a 49-year-old woman who presented following a bicycle accident with subsequent epistaxis, periorbital edema, ecchymosis, and trismus. Physical examination revealed a palpable step off over the left zygomatic arch, left malar flattening, and CN V2 distribution hypesthesia. A CT maxillofacial showed a left ZMC fracture. (*C* and *D*) Postoperative photographs 1 month following open reduction internal fixation of the left ZMC fracture. (*Courtesy of* Sunthosh Sivam, MD, Houston.)

medial canthus, and shortened palpebral fissure, is associated with naso–orbital–ethmoid (NOE) fractures. Malar depression, best assessed from a bird's eye or base view, would suggest a ZMC fracture (see **Figs. 3** and **4**). Intraoral lacerations may point toward underlying fractures of the maxilla or mandible in those areas. Similarly, deviations of the jaw with the opening of the mouth or malocclusion would also suggest a mandible fracture.

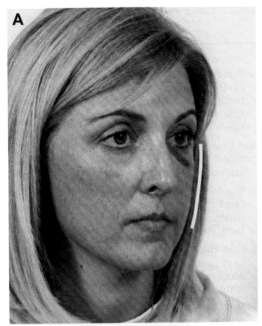

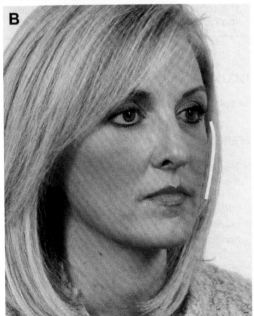

Fig. 4. (*A*) Preoperative and (*B*) postoperative oblique views highlighting interval improvement in malar projection and contour following the reduction of the patient's left ZMC fracture.

Neck Examination

Neck injuries are separated into 3 zones, which are important to keep in mind when evaluating an athlete with a cervical injury. Zone I extends from the clavicle to the cricoid cartilage, zone II from the cricoid cartilage to the angle of the mandible, and zone III from the angle of the mandible to the base of the skull. In general, vascular injuries of zone I and zone III are more difficult to control. A universal algorithm does not exist for the evaluation and treatment of neck injuries. However, physical examination has proven to be the best screening tool for injury to structures in the neck.[25]

We limit our discussion of the indications of surgical exploration as these mostly pertain to penetrating trauma to the neck. Athletic injuries are more commonly associated with blunt trauma patterns. Blunt trauma may result in symptoms of hoarseness, dyspnea, and dysphagia, suggesting injury to the aerodigestive tract, which may need urgent surgical intervention.

IMAGING

CT scans have become the gold standard for the radiographic evaluation of patients with facial

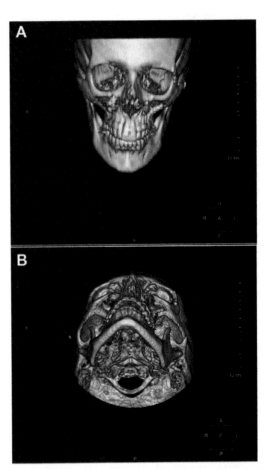

Fig. 5. Three-dimensional reconstruction of patient's postoperative CT scan illustrating interval hardware placement over the left maxilla and lateral orbital rim, with improved midface contour. (*A*) Frontal view, (*B*) Base view.

trauma, especially because of the advent of high-resolution technology and three-dimensional reconstruction (see **Fig. 5**).[9] Holmgren and colleagues showed that 12% of patients with trauma undergoing a head CT had an underlying facial fracture, with 6% having multiple fractures.[26] Therefore, an initial CT study should extend from the apex of the skull to include the inferior border of the mandible. A high-resolution scan consisting of axial cuts that are less than 1 mm in thickness allows for the accurate identification of fracture patterns as well as comprehensive surgical planning.[27]

CT angiography is predominantly reserved for the evaluation of arterial injury in the setting of penetrating neck trauma, and even in this circumstance its use still remains controversial today. Given that the incidence of penetrating trauma to the head or neck in the sports setting is very rare, CT angiography does not have a routine role in the evaluation of athletes.

Magnetic resonance imaging (MRI) may play a role in the evaluation of CNS injury or orbital injury. However, there is no routine indication for MRI to evaluate maxillofacial trauma.

SUMMARY

Sports-related injuries to the head and neck are common, and epidemiologic studies have shown that incidence has continued to increase over time.[3,4] In recent decades, regulations on violent play and protective equipment have come to the forefront in the prevention of sports-related injuries. It has been shown that players using faceguards are 35% less likely to incur facial injury than those who do not. The US Center for Disease Control and Prevention advocates for helmet use to reduce head injury, and the American Academy for Sports Dentistry lists 40 sports for which the use of mouthguards is recommended.[3,28] Encouraging usage of protective equipment is the first of many steps in reducing sports-related morbidity and mortality.

Maxillofacial trauma does not always occur in isolation, and adhering to the "ABC's" of trauma prioritizes problems that would need to be addressed in a more urgent manner, with airway being the most important. After stabilizing the patient, practitioners should use a systematic and reproducible algorithm that works consistently in evaluating patients so that injuries are not missed. The management of patients with maxillofacial trauma involves a multidisciplinary approach and coordination of care between the facial plastic surgeon, the emergency medicine physician, and any other consulting services.

CLINICS CARE POINTS

- Adhering to Advanced Trauma Life Support (ATLS) guidelines with an emphasis on airway, breathing, and circulation is critical to the safe and systematic management of all patients with facial trauma.

- A thorough head and neck examination combined with CT imaging can delineate most athletic injuries.

- The location of facial lacerations should be carefully considered for risk to underlying structures including the parotid duct and facial nerve.

- Firm digital pressure and topical decongestant sprays are the first-line treatments for acute epistaxis, followed by nasal packing materials if indicated.

- Septal and auricular hematomas should be promptly evacuated and bolstered to prevent the subsequent deformation of the underlying cartilage due to necrosis.

DISCLOSURE

The authors have nothing to disclose.

REFERENCES

1. Nam AJ, Davidson EH, Manson PN. 1.1 - assessment of the patient with traumatic facial injury. Elsevier Inc; 2020.

2. Elhammali N, Bremerich A, Rustemeyer J. Demographical and clinical aspects of sports-related maxillofacial and skull base fractures in hospitalized patients. Int J Oral Maxillofac Surg 2010;39(9): 857–62.

3. Hwang K, You SH, Lee HS. Outcome analysis of sports-related multiple facial fractures. J Craniofac Surg 2009;20(3):825–9.

4. Roccia F, Diaspro A, Nasi A, et al. Management of sport-related maxillofacial injuries. J Craniofac Surg 2008;19(2):377–82.

5. Leinhart J, Toldi J, Tennison M. Facial trauma in sports. Curr Sports Med Rep 2017;16(1):23–9.

6. Perry M. Advanced Trauma Life Support (ATLS) and facial trauma: can one size fit all?. Part 1: Dilemmas in the management of the multiply injured patient with coexisting facial injuries. Int J Oral Maxillofac Surg 2008;37(3):209–14.

7. Fonseca RJ, Allen S, Awad MK, et al. Initial assessment and intensive care of the trauma patient. 4th edition. St. Louis, Missouri: Elsevier Inc.; 2013.

8. Brooks A, Holroyd B, Riley B. Missed injury in major trauma patients. Injury 2004;35(4):407–10.

9. Chukwulebe S, Hogrefe C. The diagnosis and management of facial bone fractures. Emerg Med Clin North Am 2019;37(1):137–51.

10. Afzelius LE, Rosén C. Facial fractures: a review of 368 cases. Int J Oral Surg 1980;9(1):25–32.

11. Viozzi CF. Maxillofacial and mandibular fractures in sports. Clin Sports Med 2017;36(2):355–68.

12. Romeo SJ, Hawley CJ, Romeo MW, et al. Sideline management of facial injuries. Curr Sports Med Rep 2007;6(3):155–61.

13. Perry M, Dancey A, Mireskandari K, et al. Emergency care in facial trauma - a maxillofacial and ophthalmic perspective. Injury 2005;36(8):875–96.

14. Boswell KA. Management of facial fractures. Emerg Med Clin North Am 2013;31(2):539–51.

15. Holley J, Jorden R. Airway management in patients with unstable cervical spine fractures. Ann Emerg Med 1989;18(11):1237–9.

16. Dhara SS. Retrograde tracheal intubation. Anaesthesia 2009;64(10):1094–104.

17. Bribriesco A, Patterson GA. Cricothyroid approach for emergency access to the airway. Thorac Surg Clin 2018;28(3):435–40.

18. Lim D, Ma BC, Parumo R, et al. Thirty years of submental intubation: a review. Int J Oral Maxillofac Surg 2018;47(9):1161–5.

19. Geeraedts LMG, Kaasjager HAH, van Vugt AB, et al. Fxsanguination in trauma: a review of diagnostics and treatment options. Injury 2009;40(1):11–20.

20. Sykes LN, Cowgill F. Management of hemorrhage from severe scalp lacerations with raney clips. Ann Emerg Med 1989;18(9):995–6.

21. Robert BT, Holtmann B. Severe epistaxis in facial fractures. Plastic and Reconstructive Surgery 1983; 71(6):770–86.

22. Stevens H. Epistaxis in the athlete. Phys Sportsmed 1988;16(12):31–40.

23. Schultz RC, Camara DL. Athletic facial injuries. JAMA 1984;252(24):3395–8.

24. Steinberg MJ, Herréra AF. Management of parotid duct injuries. Oral Surg Oral Med Oral Pathol Oral Radiol Endod 2005;99(2):136–41.

25. Azuaje RE, Jacobson LE, Glover J, et al. Reliability of physical examination as a predictor of vascular injury after penetrating neck trauma. Am Surg 2003;69(9):804–7.

26. Holmgren EP, Dierks EJ, Homer LD, et al. Facial computed tomography use in trauma patients who require a head computed tomogram. J Oral Maxillofac Surg 2004;62(8):913–8.

27. Hollier LH, Sharabi SE, Koshy JC, et al. Facial trauma: general principles of management. J Craniofac Surg 2010;21(4):1051–3.

28. Exadaktylos AK, Eggensperger NM, Eggli S, et al. Sports related maxillofacial injuries: The first maxillofacial trauma database in Switzerland. Br J Sports Med 2004;38(6):750–3.

Concussion in Head Trauma

Vincent H. Key, MD[a],*, Joseph B. Noland, MD[b,1]

KEYWORDS

- Concussion • Traumatic brain injury • Sport concussion assessment tool (SCAT)
- Modified balance error scoring system (mBESS)

KEY POINTS

- Understanding that concussion or transient traumatic brain injury is multifactorial.
- The clinical manifestations of a concussion can be delayed in onset.
- Serial assessment of the patient for a concussion is critical for diagnosis and prompt treatment.
- Using the Sports Concussion Assessment Tool is important to establish a baseline and a tool to assess possible return to activity.

CONCUSSION IN THE ATHLETE AND RETURN-TO-PLAY GUIDELINES

Concussion can be a challenging diagnosis to make owing to a lack of objective binary data, often relying on self-reported history and symptoms that may be confused with or even overlap with other diagnoses. Concussion and mild or transient traumatic brain injury (tTBI) are terms that are multifaceted and multifactorial. These terms are often applied to a constellation of scenarios ranging from low-velocity occurrences (eg, running into a door) to high-impact events like car accidents and sporting injuries. The etiology is a spectrum of energy and ultimately inertia that affect the brain. Major trauma such as car accidents are probably the single most common cause of concussion. A high index of suspicion is critical to proper management of concussions. It is easy to overlook a trauma patient's head injury, especially if there are no obvious cuts or abrasions in that area. Physicians evaluating trauma patients must avoid tunnel vision that focuses only on outwardly visible injuries to the body. After stabilization of the patient, starting with the ABCs (airway, breathing, and circulation), a comprehensive secondary survey should include an assessment for acute brain injuries.

An accurate initial neurologic evaluation of the patient can be challenging in the face of multiple injuries. Many patients with tTBI do not have loss of consciousness or acute neurologic deficits. In the assessment phase of these patients, multiple serial neurologic assessments of these patients are critical. Brain injury can be ever evolving. One of the first components of the evaluation will be assessing the patient's cognitive function. Multiple neuropsychological tests are useful for this assessment.

Recognition of a patient's concussion or tTBI is crucial so that treatment that is focused on directed therapy may be started. The severity of brain injuries varies; likewise, there are differing manifestations of symptoms. The definition of concussion has gone through extensive analyses. A central question is whether concussion lies on the TBI continuum, but is associated with lesser diffuse structural changes than seen in more severe TBI. Alternatively, concussion could be a distinct entity occurring only owing to reversible physiologic changes.[1] The consensus statement on concussion in sport in Berlin (October 2016) has given the following definition of a sport-related concussion.

1. A direct cause by either a direct blow to the head, face, neck, or elsewhere on the body with an impulsive force transmitted to the head.
2. A rapid onset of short-lived impairment of neurologic function that resolves spontaneously.

[a] Orthopaedic Surgery/Sports Medicine, University of Kansas Health System, 3901 Rainbow Boulevard. Kansas City, KS 66160, USA; [b] Family Medicine, University of Kansas Health System, Kansas City, KS, USA
[1] Present address: 7405 Renner Road. Shawnee, KS 66217.
* Corresponding author.
E-mail address: vkey@kumc.edu

Facial Plast Surg Clin N Am 30 (2022) 11–14
https://doi.org/10.1016/j.fsc.2021.08.013

3. A concussion can cause neuropathological changes, but the acute clinical signs and symptoms largely reflect a functional disturbance rather than a structural injury and, as such, no abnormality is seen on standard structural neuroimaging studies.

4. A concussion results in various clinical signs and symptoms that may or may not involve a loss of consciousness. The resolution of symptoms (clinical or cognitive) typically follow a sequential course whether short or prolonged.

This challenging diagnosis can become even more difficult in the athlete population because additional obstacles are frequently present. Athletes may be motivated to not report the event and/or be unwilling to fully describe the symptoms so they can continue to play.[2] To counter these challenges, it is important to keep the patient history and physical examination consistent and standardized as much as possible. Several groups across multiple sports agree that concussion guidelines and protocols should have consistent basic principles that are adhered to, but should also be flexible enough to adapt for the particular sport and level of sport.[3] One of several tools available is the Sport Concussion Assessment Tool, 5th edition (SCAT-5). The SCAT-5 was developed in 2017 after the Berlin Concussion in Sport Consensus meeting. The SCAT-5 is designed to be used by medical professionals as an aid in diagnosing and later monitoring the progress of recovery from a concussion.[4]

In the initial evaluation of concussion, it is important to understand that a concussion is an evolving event. The evolution is based on multiple factors, such as prior injury, location of the head impact, the velocity of the head impact, and the kinematics of the brain on impact within the skull. These factors are important in terms of the acute phase of traumatic brain injury and the subsequent evaluation of the patient hours and days after injury. Unfortunately, there are no definitive tests or markers to validate the grade of the injury or to predict short or long term outcomes after the injury.

A tTBI is typically caused by a rapid acceleration/deceleration of the brain by a blow or mechanical force that causes disruption of the cell membrane and axonal integrity, triggering a complicated molecular cascade. Although a direct blow to the head can cause an tTBI, it is not the only mechanism of action to look for.[5] It is this disruption at the cellular level that accounts for the signs and symptoms of concussion. This cascade is not fully understood or delineated currently, but in the future a better understanding of the molecular processes involved could provide breakthroughs in diagnosis, prognosis, and differentiating between tTBI and more complicated diagnoses. Universally accepted criteria for the diagnosis are still not present, but all stakeholders agree that recognition and early removal from harmful situations and environments is essential for the athlete to return to normal health.[2] Some sports and sporting organizations employ a spotter who is trained to monitor for events that may cause an tTBI and to recognize signs and symptoms of an altered mental status. Regardless of whether there is a dedicated spotter or not, all coaches, staff, and players need to be educated on the signs and symptoms of tTBI. They must also feel the freedom to point these signs and symptoms out during practices and games.[2]

Once a potential mechanism of injury has been identified, the athlete should be evaluated for any red flag signs or symptoms that may indicate a need for transportation to a medical facility for emergent care. This process may include findings of double vision, seizure, increasing headache, vomiting, neck pain, or weakness in the legs and arms. This list is not a complete list of signs or symptoms that should be monitored and no list can replace sound medical decision-making after a thorough evaluation of the entire situation and circumstances.

After the athlete's immediate safety is ensured, the medical team can proceed with additional evaluation for tTBI. The mainstay of tTBI diagnosis and subsequent follow-up is evaluating signs and symptoms. To maintain standardization, a list of symptoms is given, and the athlete is asked to rate the severity of the symptom instead of providing a simple yes or no response. The athlete, not the evaluator, should be the one to fill out the checklist, including to give a severity score. In addition to being a part of the diagnostic process, the symptom score can be used to track progress throughout the recovery.[4] Although further studies need to be done, some symptoms can be predictive of timeline to return to activity.[2] It is also important to remember that signs and symptoms of tTBI can and often do evolve over time, so repeat questioning can be a valuable part of the history.

An evaluation of cognitive abilities is also important in making the diagnosis of tTBI. The evaluator has multiple areas that can be tested to assess cognition, including orientation, concentration, and immediate memory. Testing of these areas should involve consistency and several trials to provide reliable results. For the SCAT-5, a list of 10 words is read by the evaluator. The athlete then repeats as many words as possible that can be recalled. Three trials are done using the same list of 10 words to get an accurate evaluation of immediate memory.

A neurologic evaluation is a critical element of the diagnosis as well. This assessment includes a physical examination as well as balance testing. The physical examination should include an evaluation of the cranial nerves, as well as a thorough head, ears, eyes, nose, and throat examination. Evaluation of the temporomandibular joint and teeth are an important aspect owing to the potential for revealing a mechanism of injury. The neck examination should involve passive and active range of motion testing, as well as palpation of the bony vertebrae and paraspinal muscles. An evaluation for nerve involvement should include Spurling's testing, also known as the maximal cervical compression test and foraminal compression test, to look for cervical radiculopathy. Upper extremity strength, gross sensation, and deep tendon reflexes should also be tested. One way to test balance is using the modified Balance Error Scoring System.[4] This test measures postural stability that is often affected in the concussed athlete. Several maneuvers are performed by the athlete, and the evaluator is looking for specific errors that may indicate a deficit.

A long list of additional special tests are available to further assist the evaluator in assessing the vestibular and oculomotor system.[2] The medical professional should decide which test is best for their situation and experience. Regardless of the test chosen, the evaluator should be able to correctly instruct the athlete on how to do the test, know what the maneuver is testing, and know what makes it a positive or negative test. Additionally, the evaluator should always use the same tests on repeat evaluations to mark progress effectively.

Saccades are a test that evaluates the ability of the athlete to move quickly between 2 targets. Two versions are typically done, horizontal and vertical. The examiner should be looking for the athlete to give indications of difficulty in doing the maneuver, including slowed speed of eye movement as the test continues. Reproduction of symptoms, such as headache and dizziness, should be recorded as well.

The Vestibular-Ocular Reflex Cancellation test is a higher-level test that evaluates the ability to inhibit vestibular-induced eye movements. This test can also be done in 2 versions, horizontal and vertical. The evaluator monitors for the athlete and notes if they are unable to complete the test owing to dizziness or balance disruption. After the test is complete, after a 10-second pause, the evaluator should inquire about provocation of symptoms like dizziness, fogginess, photophobia, and headaches.

Currently, imaging is not beneficial in diagnosing tTBI. Research is ongoing to find ways to reliably implement advanced MRIs, but no clear role has been identified to this point. Biomarkers are another area that researchers and laboratories are investigating as an aid for diagnosis and prognosis, but no role or protocol has yet been determined.[2]

Challenges are not limited to the recognition of the inciting event, performing an accurate history and physical examination, and recording a symptom score. Additional challenges exist with making the formal diagnosis once data from tools like the SCAT-5 are combined with the physical examination and other test results. After the complete evaluation has been done, a tTBI is either diagnosed, is ruled, out or is considered to be indeterminate. If the diagnosis is made or testing is indeterminate, the athlete should be removed from play to the sideline, bench, or dugout.

The initial evaluation entails recognizing the injury, evaluating cranial nerve function, and assessing symptoms, cognitive function, behavioral signs, and balance. Multiple evaluations are usually necessary because of the possibility that symptoms may arise later. For reevaluation of the patient, the consensus statement on sports concussion in sport in Berlin (October 2016) (5) mentioned 3 key features.

a. A medical assessment including a comprehensive history and detailed neurologic examination including a thorough assessment of mental status, cognitive functioning, sleep/wake disturbance, ocular function, vestibular function, gait, and balance.
b. Determination of the clinical status of the patient, including whether there has been improvement or deterioration since the time of injury. This assessment may involve seeking additional information from parents, coaches, teammates, and eyewitnesses to the injury.
c. Determination of the need for emergent neuroimaging to exclude a more severe brain injury (eg, structural abnormality).

The treatment of patients with tTBI is multifaceted. The 4 Rs (rest, rehabilitation, refer, and recovery) are important. Rest has been controversial. Most agree that rest is important in the acute phase, although there is no solid evidence that rest will shorten the acute phase of recovery or lead to significantly better outcomes. Rehabilitation has been evolving as a critical component to concussion recovery. Cervical spine therapy along with vestibular therapy have been increasing used in the treatment algorithm of these patients with concussion. Patients with persistent symptoms after initial evaluation for a concussion (>14 days in adults and <4 weeks in children) require extra scrutiny and a more thorough evaluation. The assessment should include a comprehensive history and focused physical evaluation. There are times where special tests may be necessary such as a graded aerobic exercise test. Tests such as an electroencephalogram, brain biomarkers, or advanced neuroimaging have not yet been shown to be efficacious or add to the diagnosis. Cognitive–behavioral therapy can also help with mood or behavioral issues. Pharmacologic therapy can be helpful as well, but should be used with caution. Although medication can help with symptoms, it can also mask or even exacerbate symptoms. Recovery is considered as a return to normal activity and functioning. The timeline is very variable. Most adults see recovery at 2 weeks. Children may take up to 4 weeks for recovery. There are very few reliable preinjury predictors of either prolonged or shortened recovery. The most consistent predictor of a slower recovery is the severity of initial head injury. Some studies in children have shown that mental health issues or a history of migraine headaches can lead to a slower recovery.

CLINICS CARE POINTS

- Physicians evaluating trauma patients must avoid tunnel vision that focuses only on outwardly visible injuries to the body. After stabilization of the patient, starting with the ABCs (airway, breathing, and circulation), a comprehensive secondary survey should include an assessment for acute brain injuries.
- In the initial evaluation of concussion, it is important to understand that a "concussion" is an evolving event.
- A tTBI is typically caused by a rapid acceleration/deceleration of the brain by a blow or mechanical force that causes disruption of the cell membrane and axonal integrity, triggering a complicated molecular cascade.
- An evaluation of cognitive and neurologic abilities is also important in making the diagnosis of tTBI.
- The 4 *Rs* (rest, rehabilitation, refer, and recovery) are important in a patient's return to baseline.
- The timeline is very variable in terms of recovery. Most adults see recovery at 2 weeks. Children may take up to 4 weeks for recovery.
- The most consistent predictor of a slower recovery is the severity of initial head injury.

DISCLOSURE

The authors have nothing to disclose.

REFERENCES

1. Consensus Statement on concussion in sport-the 5th international conference on concussion in sport held in Berlin, October 2016. McCrory P, et al. Br J Sports Med 2018;51:838–47.

2. Gregory A, Poddar S. Diagnosis and Sideline management of Sport-Related Concussion. Clin Sports Med 2021;40:53–63.

3. Davis GA, Makdissi M, Bloomfield P, et al. Concussion Guidelines in Nation and International Professional and Elite Sports. Neurosurgery 2020;87(2):418–25.

4. Patricios JS, Ardern CL, Hislop MD, et al. Implementation of the 2017 Berlin Concussion in Sport Group consensus statement in contact and collision sports: a joint statement from 11 national and international sports organizations. Br J Sports Med 2018;52(10):635–41.

5. Silverberg ND, Iaccarino MA, Panenka WJ, et al. Management of Concussion and Mild Traumatic Brain Injury: A Synthesis of Practice Guidelines. Arch Phys Med Rehabil 2020;101:382–93.

Soft Tissue Injuries Including Auricular Hematoma Management

Zachary A. Zimmerman, MD*, Douglas M. Sidle, MD

KEYWORDS

- Facial trauma • Facial laceration • Dog bite • Auricular hematoma • Facial wound care
- Scar revision

KEY POINTS

- Adequate preparation and timely treatment of facial wounds is integral for an adequate functional and cosmetic result.
- Understanding surgical pearls for each specific facial subunit will help avoid pitfalls and poor results when planning and repairing facial soft tissue trauma.
- Otolaryngologist referral and management of auricular hematomas is essential to avoiding recurrence and complications such as cauliflower ear.
- The best scar revision techniques are not as efficient as initial injury repair with the eversion of skin edges, avoiding tension on the wound, lining up key landmarks, and closing the wound in layers.

INTRODUCTION

Facial trauma is among the most common craniofacial chief complaints encountered in emergency departments every year in the United States. These incidents account for nearly 7% to 10% of all emergency department visits annually.[1,2] Although the leading cause of facial soft tissue trauma is motor vehicle accidents, other causes include athletics, industrial accidents, self-inflicted trauma, falls, assault, and bites.[3,4] This population accounts for nearly 150,000 visits per year in emergency departments across the United States.[3,4] The complexity of facial soft tissue repair arises from its many functional and aesthetic subunits and the long-lasting implications related to a patient's countenance.[5]

Initially, patients with facial trauma should be evaluated for life-threatening injuries following Advance Trauma Life Support Guidelines, as facial soft tissue trauma can cause significant bleeding, potential airway compromise, or significant vascular injury.[6]

HISTORY/INITIAL EVALUATION

When evaluating facial injuries, the history of the injury and mechanism is integral to successful repair. Mechanisms such as falls, motor vehicle accidents, or gunshot wounds necessitate thorough examination for foreign material since foreign bodies impair wound healing.[7] Bite injuries increase the risk of infection due to their polymicrobial nature and may require prophylactic antibiotics or tetanus prophylaxis.[8] A visibly infected wound, usually from delayed presentation, will require therapeutic antibiotics, often directed by a culture. Prophylactic antibiotics are reserved for bite wounds or wounds with foreign material exposure and are not indicated for clean injuries.[8,9] Tetanus prophylaxis with a diphtheria-tetanus booster is indicated in those with a clean/minor wound and unknown tetanus history or less than 3 doses. In tetanus prone wounds, unknown/under vaccinated individuals receive both the booster and tetanus immunoglobulin. Tetanus prone wounds include bite wounds/punctures,

Northwestern-Department of Head and Neck Surgery, Division of Facial Plastic and Reconstructive Surgery, 675 North St Clair Street, Suite 15-200, Chicago, IL 60611, USA
* Corresponding author.
E-mail address: zazimmerman@gmail.com

Facial Plast Surg Clin N Am 30 (2022) 15–22
https://doi.org/10.1016/j.fsc.2021.08.011
1064-7406/22/© 2021 Elsevier Inc. All rights reserved.

presence of significant devitalized tissues, burns, associated sepsis, contact with soil/manure, or delayed surgical intervention (past 6 hours). Those with 3 or more doses that are up to date with boosters receive no prophylaxis in clean wounds. If they are not up to date with boosters, patients with dirty wounds receive tetanus immunoglobulin.[10] The patient's complete past medical history should be obtained. A history of diabetes, radiation therapy, alcohol abuse, or smoking has been shown to inhibit wound healing and should be noted.[3,11] Preoperative photographs and inquiring about prior craniofacial surgeries or functional deficits help restore the patient to premorbid status and set realistic expectations.[11] The use of blood thinners or medications that inhibit healing such as immunosuppressives should also be noted.

PHYSICAL EXAMINATION

Following the history, a thorough physical examination is integral. Serious injuries should be addressed before focusing on the wound and reconstructive plan. Ophthalmologic injuries or visual changes require urgent ophthalmology consultation. CT imaging should be obtained if malocclusion, palpable fracture lines, or structural instability is noted.[4] Mental status should also be assessed. One study found that with any element of impaired consciousness, an age greater than 60 years, or symptoms including headache, nausea, and vomiting, CT imaging of the brain is necessary due to the higher likelihood of a concomitant neurologic/brain injury.[12,13]

After the initial survey and physical examination, the soft tissue injuries are analyzed. The facial nerve, trigeminal nerve, and parotid duct (PD) integrity should be confirmed. If the patient is conscious, a House-Brackman score of 1 to 6 should be documented and laterality noted. More specifically, the upper, middle, and lower divisions of the nerve should all be documented separately to help localize the injury. **Fig. 1** depicts danger zones of the face that should increase suspicion for possible structural damage that may need repair. In the absence of an injury to these specific areas, paralysis or paresis could be due to edema. Complete and immediate paralysis of an area of the face coupled with a penetrating injury dictates immediate operative room repair.[14] Immediate repair in such a scenario is easier than delayed repair. The distal nerve ends can often be stimulated with a nerve stimulator, and a neurorrhaphy can be performed after devitalized edges are trimmed. If there is minimal tension at closure, primary neurorrhaphy can be performed in an epineural or perineural fashion with the aid of

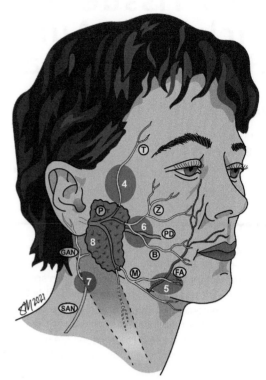

Fig. 1. Facial nerve danger zones. The temporal branch (T) of the facial nerve where it crosses the zygoma. The marginal mandibular (M) nerve where the superficial musculoaponeurotic system is thinned in the lower face. The parotid duct (PD) and the buccal (B) and zygomatic (Z) branches at the anterior border of the masseter muscle. The great auricular nerve (GAN) and the spinal accessory nerve (SAN) at Erb point on the posterior margin of the sternocleidomastoid muscle. The parenchyma of the parotid gland (P). These areas of common injury are labeled 4 to 8, respectively.

microscopy with similar outcomes.[15] This is usually performed with a monofilament, permanent, 8:0 to 10:0 suture. An interposition graft from the great auricular nerve (7 cm of length) or sural nerve (30 cm of length) has similar outcomes to primary neurorrhaphy.[14] Because both are afferent nerves, the polarization should be marked and reversed for reconstruction. Facial nerve injuries distal to a vertical line drawn from the lateral canthus often do not need to be repaired due to anastomotic branches; however, the marginal mandibular branch and temporal branch have little crossover and intervention should be considered.

After facial nerve injury has been ruled out, the wound should be inspected for saliva. As seen in **Fig. 1**, the PD travels 1.5 cm below the zygomatic arch, travels with the buccal branch of the facial nerve, turns medially at the border of the masseter, transverses the buccinator muscle, and eventually enters the oral cavity in the buccal mucosa adjacent to the second maxillary molar.[16] If saliva is present in the form of bubbles or viscous fluid, a direct parotid injury could be present opposed to an injury to stensen duct. The distal end of the duct can be located intraorally and a small 22-gauge silastic stent can be placed to locate the tear in the duct or proximal end if suspected. This can be repaired over the stent with a nonabsorbable 4:0 or 5:0 suture; the stent can be sutured to the buccal mucosa and can be removed at 2 weeks. Alternatively, if this cannot be accomplished the proximal duct can be reimplanted into the oral cavity and/or can be ligated. More commonly, saliva present in a wound signifies a parotid gland injury that can be oversewn with a braided absorbable suture and treated with conservative management with a pressure dressing. Despite the aforementioned treatments, literature shows that conservative management is generally well tolerated, and immediate surgical repair is often unnecessary.[13,17] If attempted, the patient should go to the operating room for repair.

WOUND INSPECTION/WOUND PREPARATION

Soft tissue trauma consists of abrasions, contusions, lacerations, and avulsions. An abrasion is a superficial skin injury and should be dressed with antibiotic ointment and covered. A contusion is a deeper ecchymosis that should be examined for underlying hematoma or bony injury. If hematoma is present this should be aspirated and or drained followed by the application of a pressure dressing. A laceration involves a tear that goes through the epidermis and or dermis including possible injuries to deeper tissues. An avulsion is injury with tissue loss. Occasionally an avulsion can be repaired with primary closure but may require grafts, local flaps, regional flaps, or free tissue transfer.

The size, depth, and wound base status including the viability of the wound edges and presence of gross contamination or infection should be investigated. If the wound has foreign bodies, traumatic tattooing, is a bite wound, or has not been repaired within 6 hours, it is considered contaminated. A dirty wound should undergo high-pressure pulsatile irrigation or bulb syringe irrigations with saline or a mixture of 50,000 units of bacitracin in 1 L of saline. This cleansing can be performed after anesthetizing the wound with local field or regional blocks. In an animal model, both bulb and high-pressure techniques are successful at lowering the bacterial load in wounds; however, high-pressure pulsatile irrigation is 3 times as effective.[18] Many practitioners irrigate all traumatic

facial wounds before repair despite literature supporting no benefit in clean facial and scalp injuries.[19] Realistically, a psi of 5 to 8 is accepted as adequate for cleansing traumatic wounds, making bulb irrigation sufficient.[20]

Following irrigation of dirty wounds, devitalized tissue and irregular wound edges can be debrided conservatively. Devitalized tissue impairs the wound's ability to heal and resist postoperative infection.[21,22] Extensive debridement can lead to tense wound closure and is often unnecessary due to the vast blood supply to the face. Although the wound should be prepped with povidone iodine or another similar agent, gently scrubbing the area with a high porous sponge has been found to be effective in decontamination and debridement of facial wounds without causing extensive tissue damage.[22]

SURGICAL CONSIDERATIONS

After the wound has been prepared and thoroughly examined, the setting of repair can be determined. Indications for operating room are as follows[13]:

- Patient tolerance
- Complex tissue rearrangement
- Wounds under significant tension
- Patient age
- Concomitant injuries such as facial fractures or airway compromise
- Poor hemostasis or major vascular injury
- Facial nerve injury requiring repair
- PD injury requiring repair
- Prolonged operative time greater than 2 hours

If the patient meets none of the aforementioned criteria and is not a young child, repair should be performed as soon as possible in the office or emergency department setting, as expediency of treatment has been linked to better cosmetic outcomes.[13,23] Anesthesia considerations are included:

- 1% lidocaine plain
  - Maximum dose 3 to 4 mg/kg
  - Rarely used because of lack of vasoconstrictive properties
  - Analgesic onset less than 2 minutes
  - Duration 1.5 to 2 hours
- Lidocaine 1% with epinephrine 1:100,000
  - Maximum dose 5 to 7 mg/kg
  - Commonly used due to vasoconstrictive properties
  - Analgesic onset less than 2 minutes
  - Vasoconstrictive onset 10 to 15 minutes
  - Duration 2 to 6 hours

- Bupivacaine 0.25%
  - Maximum dose 2.5 mg/kg
  - Analgesic onset less than 2 minutes
  - Duration 2 to 4 hours
- Ketamine
  - Often used in pediatric populations in the emergency department
- EMLA (eutectic mixture of local anesthetics) cream
  - Often used in the pediatric population to limit the need for local infiltration
  - Found to decrease the need for local anesthesia infiltration by 85% in extremity laceration repair[22]
- Monitored anesthesia care
  - Propofol
  - Versed and fentanyl
  - Used for shorter complex repair
- General anesthesia
  - Reserved for longer, complex repairs involving deeper or concomitant injuries

Many avoid the use of lidocaine with epinephrine in areas such as the ear and the nose for fear of necrosis and tissue compromise. The evidence supporting such complications is anecdotal and as long an intravascular injection is avoided, vasoconstrictive agents are safe in any area of the face, scalp, and neck.[24] Regional blocks should be used for larger injuries and avoid tissue distortion; however, they do not provide sufficient local vasoconstriction. Local field blocks are superior for smaller lacerations or injuries, especially when hemostasis is a major concern as in most areas of the face.[13]

SURGICAL TECHNIQUE

For an aesthetically satisfactory result, there are many key principles that should be followed for laceration repair. These key principles are listed here. Specific considerations are addressed in each facial subunit section.

- Generously undermine surrounding tissues to avoid trap door deformity from lymphatic disruption.
- Gently handle tissues with skin hooks and toothed forceps to avoid crush injury.
- Minimize tension with layered closure. Approximate the wound with absorbable inverted suture material deep (3–4:0 Monocryl, PDS, or Vicryl).
- Mucosal injuries should be closed with 3 to 5:0 absorbable suture (chromic).
- Permanent 5 to 6:0 nylon or prolene on the epidermis.

- Avoid complex repair, at least initially, if primary closure will suffice.
- Ensure adequate eversion of skin edges to avoid step-offs.
- Consider vertical mattress suture technique when eversion is difficult.
- Skin sutures should line up epidermis without strangulating the wound edges to avoid track marking.
- Long lacerations can be closed in running fashion; shorter lacerations can be closed with simple interrupted sutures.
- Consider subcuticular closure or absorbable sutures for superficial closure in children to avoid suture removal.

PERIOPERATIVE/POSTOPERATIVE MANAGEMENT

Antibiotics in the perioperative/postoperative period should be considered for mucosal wounds; contaminated wounds; bite wounds; delayed closure; and in patients with diabetes, immunocompromise, alcoholism, malnutrition, smoking, or other factors known to affect wound healing.[13] Anaerobic coverage is necessary for bite wounds. A period of 7 days is usually adequate. Keeping the epidermal layer closure clean of crusts with hydrogen peroxide and moist with antibiotic ointment has been shown to improve/expedite wound healing.[25] Patients with allergies to topical antibiotics can apply petroleum jelly–based products, and this is equally effective to antibiotic ointment.[4] Sutures are generally removed in 5 to 7 days.

SPECIAL CONSIDERATIONS BY FACIAL SUBUNIT

The following sections discuss general principles for each facial subunit as well as surgical pearls.

Scalp/Forehead

- Layers of scalp from superficial to deep: skin, connective tissue, aponeurotic tissue (galea), loose areolar tissue, pericranium
- Scalp defects less than 3 cm can generally be closed primarily but might require galeotomies.
- When closing scalp defects, layered closure is important to avoid wound dehiscence and excessive tension.
- Deep-layered closure should include a generous bite of galea.
- In the case of a large defect that cannot be closed primarily or with rotational flaps, if pericranium is intact, a skin graft can be used in non–hair-bearing scalp.

- Local pericranial, galeal, or temporoparietal fascia flaps can be used to provide a vascularized surface for a skin graft.
- Tissue expansion should not be the initial intervention in an open scalp wound but can be used secondarily for better cosmesis.
- Forehead repair can usually be accomplished primarily or with local flaps.
- If the defect is too large, a skin graft can be a temporary patch for tissue expansion but often gives unsatisfactory long-term cosmetic when used alone.

Ear

- Aside from a partial or complete avulsion, the ear can usually be repaired bedside.
- Layered closure
  - Cartilage should be approximated with a clear 4:0 PDS.
  - Anterior or visible lacerations should be closed with 5:0 prolene or nylon.
  - Posterior or hidden lacerations can be closed with absorbable suture.
- All cartilage should be covered.
- If perichondrium is exposed with skin loss, consider postauricular skin grafting from the other ear.
- Small avulsions can be reattached; total avulsions should be microsurgically repaired using superficial temporal artery or postauricular artery.[26]
  - The cartilage banking technique should be avoided and is often unsuccessful.[26]
- Although most surgeons use fluoroquinolone antibiotics for cartilage exposure to cover for pseudomonas, this practice is anecdotal and not supported by data.[27]
- Bolstering with dental rolls or mattress suturing should be performed to avoid hematoma or fluid accumulation.
- Permanent sutures and bolsters can be removed in 5 to 7 days.

Special Consideration: Auricular Hematoma Management

- Shearing forces between the perichondrium and skin can cause auricular hematomas.
- These should be drained with sterile technique to avoid cauliflower ear.
- If the hematoma or fluid collection is greater than 48 hours old or recurrent, these authors have found that scraping the area with sterile gauze after drainage can help prevent reoccurrence.
- Auricular hematomas most often occur in young men in combat sports.[28]

- Both an otolaryngology consult and a bolster dressing application have been found to prevent recurrence[28] (**Fig. 2**).

Eyelid

- Always consider an ophthalmology or oculoplastics consult if the injury is severe.
- Medial canthus injuries can cause lacrimal duct dysfunction.
- Lateral canthus injuries might require canthopexy.
- Repaired in layers of conjunctivae, tarsus/muscle, and skin.
- Upper lid injuries should be inspected for levator palpebrae disruption and repaired.
- If lid margin is involved, gray line is approximated, then muscle, then conjunctiva, and then skin.
- 6:0 to 7:0 permanent suture on skin, 4:0 to 5:0 absorbable subcutaneous sutures.
- If avulsion or tissue loss greater than 33% of upper or 50% of lower lid, consider various eyelid flaps, that is, Tezel, Hughes, Cutler-Beard flaps and so forth.

Cheek

- Usually cheek can be closed primarily due to abundance of tissue and skin laxity.
- Local flaps are preferred over full-thickness skin grafts due to poor texture and color match.

Nose

- Traditional teaching dictates that if 50% of a nasal subunit is destroyed, the remainder should be excised and the subunit should be completely reconstructed.
- Recent literature suggests disregarding this philosophy in lieu of maintaining as much tissue as possible.[29]
- If cartilage components are missing, consider auricular or rib cartilage grafts.
- Local and regional flaps can also be used for reconstruction if primary closure is not possible.
- The tip and alar rim are difficult areas to reconstruct due to the stiffness and thick skin quality.
- Functional concerns, especially in the external nasal valve area, showed be balanced with aesthetics.
- Auricular composite grafts can be used when cartilage and internal or external skin are absent.

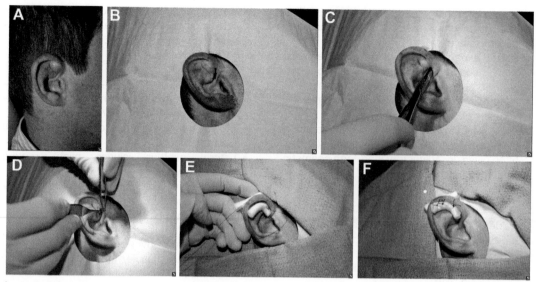

Fig. 2. Step-by-step auricular hematoma drainage and bolster. (*A*) Small auricular hematoma near root of helix. (*B*) Area prepped with betadine and 1 cm cosmetic incision marked under fold near root of helix. (*C*) After incision with number 11 blade, hemostat used to dissect pocket and ensure adequate drainage. (*D*) Small postincision pocket shown. (*E*) Bolster with dental rolls placed with 3-0 nylon mattress suture. (*F*) Bolster dressing.

- Full-thickness skin grafts can also be used rather than local flaps or primary closure but are aesthetically inferior.
- Always rule out septal hematoma, which requires incision, drainage, and splinting to avoid chondronecrosis and nasal collapse.

Lip

- Lining up lip landmarks is the key to aesthetic success, that is, vermilion border, Cupid's bow, and philtral columns.
- Mark key landmarks before distortion/injection with local.
- If less than on-third of the lip is missing, primary closure usually is achievable.
- The vermillion border should be approximated first with a superficial suture.
- Edges should be debrided, cleaned, and the defect crafted into a wedge, if possible, for better aesthetic result.

- Key stitch should approximate the vermillion, and this is the first suture placed.
- The orbicularis layer is closed with 4:0 braided suture, the mucosa is then closed with 4:0 chromic suture, and the skin with 5:0 permanent monofilament.
- Lip flaps for defects over 33% of lip
  - Abbe flap used for up to 50% of lip not involving commissure
  - Estlander flap used for up to 50% of lip involving commissure
  - Bernard-Webster, Gillies fan flap, Karapandzic flap, and Nakajima flap used for larger defects

Bite Wounds

Nearly 90% of bite wounds presenting to the emergency department in the United States are due to dogs. As aforementioned, tetanus and rabies status should be queried and treated

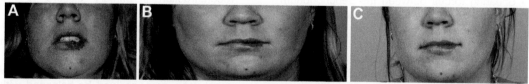

Fig. 3. A dog bite wound of the lower lip with tissue avulsion and loss, which was treated within 8 hours of presentation. (*A*) Initial wound involving mucosal lip, red lip, and vermilion border. (*B*) Six weeks postrepair with mucosal advancement with abdominal dermal fat graft. Specifically note the volume loss and oral incompetence. (*C*) Six weeks postrevision 1 year after the initial repair with abdominal fat harvest and injection of 1.5 mL into the left lower lip.

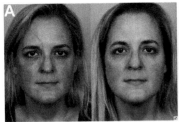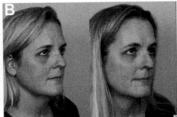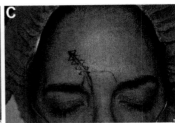

Fig. 4. A well-healed laceration of the glabella/forehead and scar revision with running W-plasty followed by dermabrasion 6 weeks afterward. (*A*) Frontal (before on left, after on right). (*B*) Three-quarters view (before on left, after on right). (*C*) Running W-plasty markings.

appropriately. A wound presenting outside of 24 hours should undergo delayed repair and a period of 4 to 5 days should be allowed to pass while treating with antibiotics until definitive closure.[8] Primary closure should be delayed in the event of active infection or late presentation. Evidence does not support the use of antibiotics for dog bite wounds but strongly suggests the use of antibiotics with cat and human bites. Despite the literature, it is reasonable to cover all bites on the face with prophylactic antibiotics for 3 to 5 days even given the low infection rate, as a facial wound infection could have deleterious cosmetic consequences.[8] The 2 most common pathogens include Pasteurella spp and Streptococcus viridans spp from animal bites and human bites, respectively. Oral anaerobes are also prevalent in bite injuries and include Fusobacterium, Prevotella, Bacteroides, and Porphyromonas spp. Empirical antibiotics of choice include amoxicillin/clavulanic acid for 3 to 5 days or doxycycline if penicillin allergic. Azithromycin is appropriate in a penicillin-allergic pregnant female and in penicillin-allergic children in which case the alternatives aforementioned are contraindicated.[8] The wounds should be debrided, thoroughly irrigated, and closed expediently (**Fig. 3**).

Scar Revision

The best facial scars result from a well-planned, layered, and intricate wound repair. After initial suture removal, silicone sheeting has been proved to aid in creating a flat and less noticeable scar.[30] It also helps avoid hypertrophic scarring and keloids. A widened or depressed scar can result from poor layered closure or excessive tension. Depending on the length and location of the scar, reexcision and closure may be an option. Z-plasty is a useful technique in contracted scars and works to lengthen the scar while blending the new scar in the relaxed skin tension lines (RSTL). The W-plasty, depicted in **Fig. 4**, reorients a shorter scar along the RSTL, making the new scar less noticeable. A geometric broken line is

useful for longer scars. Formal scar revision/excision should not take place for up to 4 to 6 months after initial repair. Often, these procedures are followed by dermabrasion for color variations or contour irregularities 6 weeks after initial repair or scar revision. Laser treatments may also improve unsatisfactory scars.

CLINICS CARE POINTS

- Ruling out other serious injuries such as neurovascular pathology or airway concerns is the first step in facial soft tissue trauma management.
- Prophylactic antibiotics are usually not necessary in clean wounds.
- Patients with comorbid conditions such as diabetes, smokers, those on immunosuppressive medications, alcohol abuse, and with a history of radiation therapy are at a higher risk for poor wound healing.
- Prompt treatment of bite wounds that show no evidence of infection and treatment with antibiotics is important for superior cosmetic results.
- If there is immediate facial paralysis, the patient should be taken to the operating room urgently for concomitant exploration and repaired to improve functional outcomes.
- Otolaryngology referral/consultation for auricular hematoma management is essential to avoid recurrence.
- Scar revision techniques such as Z-plasty, W-plasty, geometric broken line closure, dermabrasion, and silicone sheeting can help alleviate irregularities from initial repair.

DISCLOSURE

The authors have nothing to disclose.

REFERENCES

1. Hussain K, Wijetunge DB, Grubnic S, et al. A comprehensive analysis of craniofacial trauma. J Trauma 1994;36(1):34–47.
2. Ong TK, Dudley M. Craniofacial trauma presenting at an adult accident and emergency department with an emphasis on soft tissue injuries. Injury 1999;30(5):357–63.
3. Hochberg J, Ardenghy M, Toledo S, et al. Soft Tissue Injuries to Face and Neck: Early Assessment and Repair. World J Surg 2001;25(8):1023–7.
4. Patel KGMDP, Sykes JMMD. Management of soft-tissue trauma to the face. Oper Tech Otolaryngol Head Neck Surg 2008;19(2):90–7.
5. Williams RY, Wohlgemuth SD. Does the "rule of nines" apply to morbidly obese burn victims? J Burn Care Res 2013;34(4):447–52.
6. Perry M, Dancey A, Mireskandari K, et al. Emergency care in facial trauma—a maxillofacial and ophthalmic perspective. Injury 2005;36(8):875–96.
7. Motamedi MH. Primary Treatment of Penetrating Injuries to the Face. J Oral Maxillofac Surg 2007;65(6):1215–8.
8. Stefanopoulos PK, Tarantzopoulou AD. Management of Facial Bite Wounds. Dent Clin North Am 2009;53(4):691–705.
9. Medel N, Panchal N, Ellis E. Postoperative Care of the Facial Laceration. Craniomaxillofac Trauma Reconstr 2010;3(4):189–200.
10. Miyagi K, Shah AK. Tetanus prophylaxis in the management of patients with acute wounds. J Plast Reconstr Aesthet Surg 2011;64(10):e267–9.
11. Braun TL, Maricevich RS. Soft Tissue Management in Facial Trauma. Semin Plast Surg 2017;31(2):073–9.
12. Ono K, Wada K, Takahara T, et al. Indications for Computed Tomography in Patients With Mild Head Injury. Neurol Med Chir 2007;47(7):291–8.
13. Kretlow JD, McKnight AJ, Izaddoost SA. Facial Soft Tissue Trauma. Semin Plast Surg 2010;24(4):348–56.
14. Gordin E, Lee TS, Ducic Y, et al. Facial Nerve Trauma: Evaluation and Considerations in Management. Craniomaxillofac Trauma Reconstr 2015;8(1):001–13.
15. Rouleau M, Crepeau J, Tetreault L, et al. Facial nerve sutures: epineural vs. perineural sutures. J Otolaryngol 1981;10(5):338–42.
16. Robardey G, Le Roux MK, Foletti JM, et al. The Stensen's duct line: A landmark in parotid duct and gland injury and surgery. A prospective anatomical, clinical and radiological study. J Stomatol Oral Maxillofac Surg 2019;120(4):337–40.
17. Lewis G, Knottenbelt JD. Parotid duct injury: is immediate surgical repair necessary? Injury 1991;22(5):407–9.
18. Svoboda MSJ, Bice TG, Gooden HA, et al. Comparison of Bulb Syringe and Pulsed Lavage Irrigation with Use of a Bioluminescent Musculoskeletal Wound Model. J Bone Joint Surg Am 2006;88(10):2167–74.
19. Hollander JE, Richman PB, Werblud M, et al. Irrigation in Facial and Scalp Lacerations: Does It Alter Outcome? Ann Emerg Med 1998;31(1):73–7.
20. Edlich RF, Rodeheaver GT, Morgan RF, et al. Principles of emergency wound management. Ann Emerg Med 1988;17(12):1284–302.
21. Haury B, Rodeheaver G, Vensko J, et al. Debridement: an essential component of traumatic wound care. Am J Surg 1978;135(2):238–42.
22. Hollander JE, Singer AJ. Laceration Management. Ann Emerg Med 1999;34(3):356–67.
23. Aveta A, Casati P. Soft tissue injuries of the face: early aesthetic reconstruction in polytrauma patients. Ann Ital Chir 2008;79(6):415–7.
24. Häfner HM, Röcken M, Breuninger H. Epinephrine-supplemented local anesthetics for ear and nose surgery: Clinical use without complications in more than 10,000 surgical procedures. J Dtsch Dermatol Ges 2005;3(3):195–9.
25. Goslen JB. Wound Healing for the Dermatologic Surgeon. J Dermatol Surg Oncol 1988;14(9):959–73.
26. Gailey AD, Farquhar D, Clark JM, et al. Auricular avulsion injuries and reattachment techniques: A systematic review. Laryngoscope Invest Otolaryngol 2020;5(3):381–9.
27. Williams CH, Sternard BT. Complex ear lacerations. Treasure Island (FL): StatPearls; 2021.
28. Dalal PJ, Purkey MR, Price CPE, et al. Risk factors for auricular hematoma and recurrence after drainage. Laryngoscope 2020;130(3):628–31.
29. Rohrich RJ, Griffin JR, Ansari M, et al. Nasal reconstruction—beyond aesthetic subunits: a 15-year review of 1334 cases. Plast Reconstr Surg (1963) 2004;114(6):1405–16.
30. Kim JS, Hong JP, Choi JW, et al. The Efficacy of a Silicone Sheet in Postoperative Scar Management. Adv Skin Wound Care 2016;29(9):414–20.

Nasal Fractures

Kelly C. Landeen, MD[a], Kyle Kimura, MD[a], Scott J. Stephan, MD[b],*

KEYWORDS

- Nasal fracture • Septal fracture • Closed reduction • Open reduction • Rhinoplasty

KEY POINTS

- Nasal bone fractures comprise >50% of all facial fractures.
- Approximately half of all nasal bone fractures will have other associated facial fractures.
- CT is the gold standard imaging modality for nasal bone fractures.
- Nasal trauma workup must include evaluation for septal hematoma.
- Displaced nasal bone fractures should undergo closed reduction within 14 days of injury if possible.

INTRODUCTION

The nose is the gateway to our respiratory system and the cornerstone of the face, giving nasal injuries the potential to be both functionally and cosmetically impactful. The central location and natural projection of the nose away from the face makes it highly susceptible to injury from sports, assaults, and motor vehicle collisions; in fact, the nasal bones are the most frequently injured bones of the face. In this article we review the evaluation and management of nasal facial trauma, including fractures of the nasal bones, septum, and nasal cartilages.

NASAL ANATOMY

Externally the nose is composed of 2 paired nasal bones that form the superior bony wall of the nasal cavity, colloquially referred to the as the nasal bridge. The bones articulate with each other in the midline, superiorly with the frontal bone, posteriorly with the perpendicular plate of the ethmoid bone, and laterally with the frontal process of the maxilla. Inferior and caudal to the nasal bones lie the paired upper lateral cartilages, which are triangular and provide shape to most of the nasal dorsum. The nasal bones articulate with the upper lateral cartilages at an area referred to as the keystone. This junction provides stability and structure of the nasal dorsum. Continuing caudal along the nose, the upper lateral cartilages articulate with the paired lower lateral cartilages at the scroll region, which is one of the major mechanisms of nasal tip support. The lower lateral cartilages curl inferomedially to shape the nasal alae, which are flanked laterally by accessory cartilage and fibrofatty tissue.

The nasal septum is a combined bony and cartilaginous structure in the midline that divides the right and left nasal cavities. It is formed by the quadrangular cartilage, the perpendicular plate of the ethmoid, the vomer, the horizontal plate of the palatine bone, and the maxillary crest. The septum also houses a diverse vascular supply with several feeding vessels contributing to this region. Along the anterior septum, Kiesselbach plexus is a confluence of arteries from branches of the sphenopalatine and facial arteries. Posteriorly, Woodruff plexus provides blood flow from the sphenopalatine and posterior pharyngeal arteries. These highly vascularized regions provide collateral blood flow and may be a source of epistaxis following nasal trauma.

TRENDS IN NASAL BONE FRACTURES

Owing to its structure and location the nose is highly susceptible to injury, and nasal bone

[a] Department of Otolaryngology–Head and Neck Surgery, Vanderbilt University Medical Center, 1215 21st Ave S7 South, Nashville, TN 37232, USA; [b] Division of Facial Plastic and Reconstructive Surgery, Department of Otolaryngology–Head and Neck Surgery, Vanderbilt University Medical Center, 1215 21st Ave S7 South, Nashville, TN 37232, USA
* Corresponding author.
E-mail address: stephan@vumc.org

Facial Plast Surg Clin N Am 30 (2022) 23–30
https://doi.org/10.1016/j.fsc.2021.08.002

fractures comprise more than 50% of all facial fractures.[1,2] Common mechanisms of injury include assault and sports-related injuries, and less commonly motor vehicle collisions. Nasal fractures occur twice as often in men as in women with some postulating that this is due to a higher male predominance in contact sports and physical altercations.[1,2]

Fracture patterns often arise based on the type of trauma. Anterior impacts result in damage to the nasal tip and cartilages, resulting in a flattened nasal dorsum and splayed nasal bones. Lateral impacts result in depressed displacement of nasal bones, C- or S-shaped nasal dorsum deformities, and medial maxillary wall fractures. Both anterior and lateral forces can lead to septal deformities. There are often associated fractures including the maxilla, orbit, and septum. As many as 67% of nasal bone fractures also have fractures of the frontal process of the maxilla, and as many as 42% have associated septal fractures (**Fig. 1**).[3]

Although classification systems for nasal bone fractures exist, none have been widely adopted by the facial trauma community. The Stranc-Robertson classification system was proposed in 1979 and stratifies injuries into three different planes based on frontal and lateral injury.[4,5] The Murray classification system from 1986 was developed by experimental injuries to cadaveric nasal bones and is based on pathologic findings and trends.[6] The Modified Murray classification was proposed in 2007 and classifies nasal bone fractures in increasing severity based on displacement, laterality, and comminution.[7] Despite these existing classification systems, clinicians instead often rely on descriptions of fractures based on examination and radiographic findings and terminology. Fractures are thus often described as unilateral or bilateral, displaced or nondisplaced, splayed, impacted, telescoped, or comminuted.

EVALUATION AND WORKUP OF NASAL FRACTURES

When working up nasal bone fractures, the initial step is to collect a thorough patient history including the nature of trauma and associated injuries, as well as evaluation for loss of consciousness, epistaxis, and perceived new-onset nasal obstruction. A thorough physical examination should be performed and any signs of epistaxis, bony step-offs, open fractures, and evidence of nasal obstruction should be noted. Examination should include anterior rhinoscopy and endonasal palpation to assess for obstruction, narrowing of the internal nasal valve, and septal hematoma. Bruising and tenderness may also serve as a clue to an underlying nasal bone fracture. Epistaxis should be managed in the acute setting, because inadequately addressed nasal bone fractures can lead to persistent epistaxis due to mucosal disruption overlying the fracture line. Nasal obstruction should be documented and followed clinically after management of the fractures. Note that swelling from the trauma may confound the evaluation and disguise or exacerbate evidence of nasal dorsal deviation or deformity. Photodocumentation is a helpful tool for assessing progression of swelling and deformity.

Although not necessarily indicated in isolated nasal bone fractures, imaging is often obtained following facial trauma to evaluate for concurrent maxillofacial bony injury. Depending on the mechanism of trauma, it may be indicated for medicolegal documentation. Lateral plain film radiographs are typically used in the acute care setting. These radiographs may definitively show nasal bone fractures but are limited in their ability to identify nondisplaced nasal bone fractures and septal injury. Noncontrasted computed tomography is much more commonly used in the emergency department setting and evaluates for nasal injury and other facial and head injuries. Although all planes should be evaluated, axial views are often the best way to evaluate for nasal bone fracture, as the axial plane best demonstrates nasal bone displacement, depression, splaying, impaction, and comminution (**Fig. 2**). Imaging may be deferred in certain settings if there is strong clinical evidence of fracture and no concern for associated injuries, or if there is low suspicion for fracture due to no obvious deformity or nasal obstruction.

COMPLICATED NASAL FRACTURES

When evaluating nasal bone fractures, one must also evaluate for other associated injuries and for complications including cosmetic and functional deformity. As previously mentioned, there may also be fractures of nearby structures such as the orbit, septum, and frontal process of the maxilla. Fractures of the pyriform aperture that are medially displaced must also be identified, because failure to reduce them may result in the medial buttress setting in such a way that causes significant nasal obstruction. Depending on the mechanism of injury, there may be more extensive facial or skull base fractures. If there are skull base fractures or injury to the cribriform plate, evaluation for cerebrospinal fluid leak and anosmia must be performed. Certain fracture patterns may also result in injury to the medial canthal

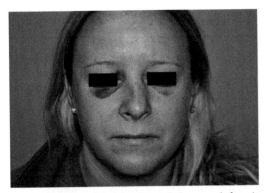

Fig. 1. Example of C-shaped nasal dorsum deformity due to right-sided impact, with medial displacement (depression) of right nasal bone and lateral displacement (widening) of left nasal bone. Note the mild surrounding ecchymosis and edema. Photograph taken 4 days after initial trauma.

ligament, leading to deformity and dysfunction of the eyelid and lacrimal duct.

Cartilaginous injury is rarer due to their flexible nature but may also be present in nasal trauma. This injury is often associated with injury of the high perpendicular plate, which affects the keystone and can cause disarticulation of the upper lateral cartilages from the nasal bones; this results in a depression of the middle third of the nose made more evident during inspiration. Nasal cartilage fracture or dislocation requires resuspension of the nasal cartilages to prevent persistent obstruction or dynamic collapse, and this often

requires operative repair with or without cartilage grafting.

One of the most common complications of nasal bone fractures is injury to the nasal septum. This injury includes septal dislocation, fracture, or hematoma. Dislocation and fracture of the septum may require reduction depending on displacement and degree of functional deficit. It should be noted that concomitant septal fractures are associated with worse functional outcome after closed nasal bone reduction and is a risk factor for future open septorhinoplasty.[8] Septal hematomas can lead to abscess formation or septal necrosis, which in turn can lead to septal perforation or a loss of the height of the nasal dorsum, known as a saddle nose deformity (**Fig. 3**). Hematomas must be evacuated, and septal splints, nasal packing, or a quilting stitch should be placed as a bolster to prevent fluid from reaccumulating.

CLOSED REDUCTION OF NASAL FRACTURES

Displaced nasal bone and septal fractures are typically managed with closed reduction, which can be effective in the appropriate setting. Closed reduction is indicated if there is visible deformity or nasal obstruction attributed to the injury; it is useful in unilateral or bilateral displaced fractures, particularly depressed fractures.[1,2] Closed reduction should not be performed if there is a cribriform plate fracture, because this puts the patient at risk for cerebrospinal fluid leak and olfactory cleft injury. In the setting of peritraumatic swelling it is

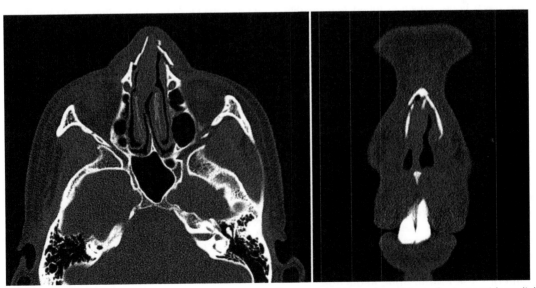

Fig. 2. Axial and coronal computed tomographic images demonstrate bilateral nasal bone fractures with medial displacement (depression) of the right nasal bone and comminution and lateral displacement of the left nasal bone. Note the associated superior septal bone fracture on the coronal image.

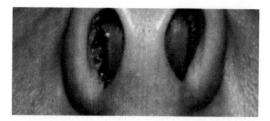

Fig. 3. Example of nasal septal hematoma on anterior rhinoscopy.

important to correlate clinical evaluation with radiographic findings of displacement.

Local Versus General Anesthesia for Closed Nasal Bone Reduction

One of the most important factors to consider in closed reduction of nasal fractures is whether these can be performed at the bedside or clinic setting under local anesthesia, or if they should be performed under general anesthesia. Some institutions have initiated image guidance for closed reduction under general anesthesia, which does improve the degree of reduction, but incurs more cost and has not been evaluated in terms of patient satisfaction.[9]

The largest benefit of bedside reduction with local anesthesia is avoidance of anesthesia, which carries its own health and cost risks; general anesthesia, however, eliminates patient discomfort and pain during the procedure and can provide the surgeon with more aggressive manipulation to ensure adequate reduction. One meta-analysis of studies comparing local versus general anesthesia for closed nasal bone reduction found that despite increased cost and risks of general anesthesia, patient satisfaction in esthetic and functional outcomes was higher in those who had received general anesthesia, and they were less likely to need secondary corrective surgery; however, only the improved esthetic outcome was statistically significant.[10]

Bedside reduction should thus only be attempted if (1) adequate reduction can reasonably be achieved and (2) the patient will tolerate the procedure, or if the patient cannot tolerate general anesthesia. If bedside reduction is attempted, the physician can make the procedure more tolerable for the patient with any combination of topical anesthetics, injectable anesthetics, nerve blocks, intranasal vasoconstrictors, anxiolytics, and systemic pain medications.

Timing of Closed Nasal Bone Reduction

The timing of closed reduction is a vital factor in management of nasal fractures. Local edema and inflammation can interfere with the ability to adequately assess nasal deformity, as well as the ability to reduce the fracture in the acute setting. Conversely, reduction should be performed before the bones have begun to heal and set incorrectly. Most literature recommends treatment within 14 days of the initial injury,[11–13] although 2 studies found that delayed repair of nasal fractures had good outcomes up to 4[14] or even 5 weeks following initial injury.[15] Regardless of the exact timing, there is a consensus among facial trauma surgeons that there exists a critical window of opportunity in which these fractures should be addressed.

- Immediate repair: Ideally performed less than 3 hours from the initial injury, before major swelling has taken place and distorted the appreciation of nasal anatomy.
- Delayed repair: Typically performed 3 to 14 days following initial injury, after edema has improved but nasal bones have not set in the posttraumatic location. Improvement in swelling may be accelerated using ice packs.

Failure to perform reduction within these time frames puts patients at greater risk for failed or inadequate reduction. These patients may ultimately require more procedures in the future, including operative procedures with osteotomies to allow for adequate bony reduction.[11–16]

Techniques for Closed Nasal Bone Reduction

Medially displaced nasal bones are typically reduced by placing a long, flat instrument such as a Boies elevator into the nare along the endonasal dorsum (**Fig. 4**). If a Boies elevator is unavailable, the broad side of a scalpel handle may be used, with the blade removed for safety. While this instrument is used to apply tension within the nare, manual pressure is applied externally to the nasal bone and, using a rocking motion, the bone is pushed back into correct alignment. For laterally displaced nasal bones, an endonasal instrument may be helpful but is not always necessary. A Killian nasal speculum may also be used to provide both endonasal and external pressure for reduction of the displaced bone.

Techniques for Closed Reduction of Septum

A fractured septum may be reduced in a similar fashion to fractured nasal bones. In this instance, Walsham or Asch forceps are the instruments of choice, because they provide pressure on both sides of the septum and can easily be placed into bilateral nares. Ultimately, the nasal septum should be straightened and repositioned centrally

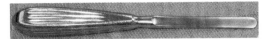

Fig. 4. Boies elevator, an endonasal instrument for nasal bone reduction.

onto the maxillary crest. Nasal endoscopy should be performed afterward to ensure complete reduction and no new-onset hematoma (**Fig. 5**).

Postprocedural Care Following Closed Reduction of Nasal Bone and Septal Fractures

After nasal fractures have been reduced, it is not uncommon for the patient to experience mild to moderate epistaxis. This epitaxis can be managed with oxymetazoline, alar pressure if tolerated, hemostatic agents, and absorbable or nonabsorbable nasal packing if it persists.

Nasal packing may assist in compression of the septum following evacuation of a septal hematoma but is used much less frequently due to increased patient discomfort and the risk of dangerous complications, including toxic shock syndrome and vagal responses such as bradycardia and hypoxia.[17] Furthermore, excessive pressure placed on septal mucosa from nonabsorbable packing may lead to septal perforation. If the nose is packed with nonabsorbable material, antibiotic prophylaxis should be considered to avoid infection and should be removed within 5 days of placement. Septal splints can be used to prevent septal hematoma and further dislocation of the septum and are typically tolerated better than packing.

An external splint or tape is often placed over the nasal dorsum following reduction to prevent repeat trauma and to remind the patient to avoid touching the nose or manipulating the nasal soft tissues; this is typically left in place for 5 to 7 days.[2] The patient should also have close clinical follow-up in this time frame to ensure adequate reduction, because patients may require further procedures in 9% to 50% of cases of nasal trauma.[2,12] All patients undergoing closed reduction must be counseled that an open septorhinoplasty may ultimately be necessary for an acceptable cosmetic and functional outcome (**Fig. 6**).

OPEN REDUCTION OF NASAL AND SEPTAL FRACTURES

In some instances, closed reduction may not sufficiently reduce nasal fractures and open reduction is indicated; this includes some greenstick fractures, which may require osteotomies to complete the fracture and allow for osseous mobilization. Similarly, telescoping comminution of nasal bones may require open reduction, because closed reduction will not be adequate and may result in areas that lack bone entirely. In these cases, small external incisions may be accessed for osteotomies and fracture manipulation.

If there is extensive soft tissue injury, damage to the keystone or scroll regions, severe septal injury, or open fractures, a primary open septorhinoplasty may be indicated. External interosseous wires or plates may also provide fixation but should be used judiciously because of the risk of skin necrosis and patient discomfort.[9,10] Open repair may also be used if there are other facial fractures that require operative repair, such as nasoorbito-ethmoidal complex or orbital floor fractures.

If closed reduction of nasal fractures is performed in the immediate or delayed postinjury period but later deemed inadequate, open septorhinoplasty may be performed weeks to months after the injury to address persistent cosmetic or

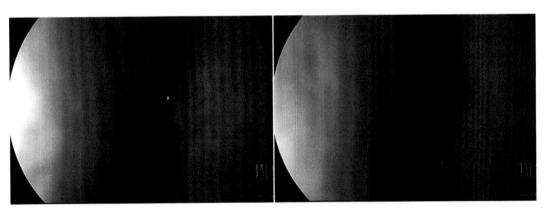

Fig. 5. Endoscopic view of left nasal bone and septal fracture, with the lateralized septum causing narrowing of the nasal cavity. The image on the right was obtained after nasal and septal reduction, with marked increase in nasal cavity size.

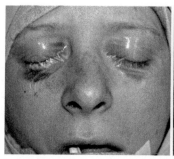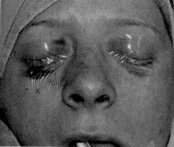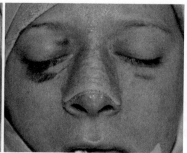

Fig. 6. Bilateral nasal bone fractures from right lateral impact before closed reduction, after closed reduction, and after placement of an external nasal splint.

functional abnormality. Patients with preinjury nasal obstruction or concurrent traumatic septal fractures are more likely to require future surgeries.[8,11,12,16,18] Open septorhinoplasty may also be performed if no interventions were performed because of the lack of perceived deformity, but the patient later identifies unacceptable cosmetic deformity or nasal obstruction.

SPECIAL CONSIDERATIONS IN PEDIATRIC NASAL TRAUMA

Nasal trauma is less common in children overall but, like in adults, is more common in males than females. Mechanisms of pediatric nasal trauma are mostly falls in young children and sports injuries in adolescents.[19] Children have a greater relative cartilaginous composition of the nose, a more rigid septum, and less overall frontal projection, all of which lead to higher likelihood of post-trauma complications after nasal trauma. Children are also more likely to have associated septal fractures, septal hematoma, and other facial fractures; they are also more likely to have greenstick or comminuted nasal bone fractures. Owing to the smaller endonasal dimensions in children, they are also at higher risk of postinjury or postprocedure synechiae and stenosis.[13]

Pediatric nasal fractures are almost always repaired due to the possible effect of unrepaired fractures on normal nasal growth. The septum undergoes bimodal growth before age 5 years and again at puberty, so age is an important factor when determining if interventions are indicated. The cartilaginous septum is a key determinant in normal growth of the nose, and septal abnormalities can lead to poor cosmesis, midface hypoplasia, and malocclusion.[20]

Special consideration, however, must be taken when considering bedside closed reduction in pediatric patients. Most children are poor candidates for bedside procedures because of poor tolerance and often require procedural sedation or general anesthesia.[13,14] General anesthesia also allows for more thorough evaluation and reduction of fractures, which can help reduce the risk of abnormal growth development.

VARIATION IN MANAGEMENT OF NASAL TRAUMA

This article discusses the overall management of nasal trauma, although it should be noted that treatment algorithms may vary significantly based on cost analysis, institution, and patient and family preferences. For example, closed reduction in the operating room may result in more successful reduction of nasal bone fractures, but the high cost of general anesthesia may be a major deterrent to the patient. Inadequate reduction, however, can lead to much greater costs in the future if an open rhinoplasty is indicated. Alternatively, a patient may be unwilling to undergo bedside procedures and will instead elect for operative interventions. Patients without transportation or poor support systems may be best managed in the acute setting rather than monitored during outpatient follow-up. Some patients may prefer no interventions despite acquired deformity or obstruction, and their wishes should be respected.

Variation has also been demonstrated in the management of patients based on provider subspecialty and training. Most nasal fractures are initially evaluated by primary care or emergency room providers and may be managed definitively in these settings, but more often nasal fractures are managed by a subspecialty-trained plastic surgeon, otolaryngologist, or oral and maxillofacial surgeon.[21] This variation in facial trauma coverage may lead to varied management algorithms and interventions. For example, otolaryngologists are more likely than plastic surgeons to evaluate for nasal obstruction, follow patients in an outpatient setting, and perform operative interventions; plastic surgeons are more likely to manage patients in an acute or inpatient setting.[22] Although no study has demonstrated a difference in overall outcomes or need for revision surgery based on subspecialty consultant, there remains no standardized treatment algorithm for management of nasal trauma. Ultimately, management of nasal trauma is determined not only by medical and surgical indications but also by patient, provider, and institution preference.

SUMMARY AND KEY POINTS

- Nasal bone fractures are the most common facial fractures in both adults and children and are more common in males.
- Nasal trauma often has associated injuries including septal and other facial fractures, septal hematoma, skull base fractures, spinal fluid leak, lacrimal duct injury, and olfactory cleft injury
- Treatment of nasal trauma is determined by the presence of cosmetic deformity and functional impairment
- Nasal bone and septal fractures are most commonly treated with closed reduction
  - Closed reduction can be performed at bedside if the patient will tolerate the procedure or may be performed under sedation or general anesthesia.
  - The best time for closed reduction is less than 3 hours from injury before swelling has set in or 3 to 14 days after injury when swelling has subsided but the bones have not set into their current position.
  - Patients with inadequate closed reduction may ultimately need an open septorhinoplasty to address cosmesis or nasal obstruction.
- Septal hematoma must be identified and managed urgently because of the risk of septal necrosis, abscess formation, and saddle nose deformity.
- Open septorhinoplasty may be performed primarily for complex, comminuted, and severely deformed nasal and septal fractures.
- Nasal cartilage fracture and dislocation are rare, but often require an open procedure with resuspension of the soft tissues.
- Special care should be taken in pediatric nasal trauma, because inadequate reduction of nasal bone and septal fractures can lead to impaired nasal growth and deformity.
- There is great variation in the evaluation and management of nasal trauma based on institution, provider, subspecialty consultant, and patient preference.

DISCLOSURE

The authors have no personal or financial conflicts of interest to disclose.

REFERENCES

1. Josh RR, Trujillo O, Koch CA, et al. Head and Neck Trauma: Nasal Fractures. In: Pasha R, Golub JS, editors. Otolaryngology – Head and Neck Surgery: Clinical Reference Guide. 6th ed. Plural Publishing, Inc; 2017. p. 658–9.
2. Kelley BP, Downey CR, Stal S. Evaluation and reduction of nasal trauma. Semin Plast Surg 2010;24(4):339–47.
3. Li L, Zang H, Han D, et al. Nasal bone fractures: analysis of 1193 cases with an emphasis on coincident adjacent fractures. Facial Plast Surg Aesthet Med 2020;22(4):249–54.
4. Stranc MF, Robertson GA. A classification of injuries of the nasal skeleton. Ann Plast Surg 1979;2(6):468–74.
5. Musculoskeletal Key. Photo of planes in Stranc classification. Available at: https://musculoskeletalkey.com/wp-content/uploads/2016/07/B9781416037729500298_f21-011-9781416037729.jpg. Accessed January 15, 2021.
6. Murray JA, Maran AG, Busuttil A, et al. A pathological classification of nasal fractures. Injury 1986;17(5):338–44.
7. Stal S, Higuera S, Lee EI, et al. Nasal trauma and the deviated nose. Plast Reconstr Surg 2007;120(7 Suppl 2):64S–75S.
8. Arnold MA, Yanik SC, Suryadevara AC. Septal fractures predict poor outcomes after closed nasal reduction: retrospective review and survey. Laryngoscope 2019;129(8):L1784–90.
9. Chung JH, Yeo HD, Yoon ES, et al. Comparison of the outcomes of closed reduction nasal bone fractures with a surgical navigation system. J Craniofac Surg 2020;31(6):1625–8.
10. Al-Moraissi EA, Ellis E III. Local versus general anesthesia for the management of nasal bone fractures: a systematic review and meta-analysis. J Oral Maxillofac Surg 2015;73(4):606–15.
11. Staffel JG. Optimizing treatment of nasal fractures. Laryngoscope 2002;112(1):1709–19.
12. Rohrich RJ, Adams WP Jr. Nasal fracture management: minimizing secondary nasal deformities. Plast Reconstr Surg 2000;106:266–73.
13. Ridder GJ, Boedeker CC, Fradis M, et al. Technique and timing for closed reduction of isolated nasal fractures: a restrospective study. Ear Nose Throat J 2002;81(1):49–54.
14. Yoon HY, Han DG. Delayed reduction of nasal bone fractures. Arch Craniofac Surg 2016;17(2):51–5.
15. Basheeth N, Donnelly M, David S, et al. Acute nasal fracture management: a prospective study and literature review. Laryngoscope 2015;125(12):2677–84.

16. Li K, Moubayed SP, Spataro E, et al. Risk factors for corrective septorhinoplasty associated with initial treatment of isolated nasal fracture. JAMA Facial Plast Surg 2018;20(6):460–7.

17. Fairbanks DN. Complications of nasal packing. Otolaryngol Head Neck Surg 1986;94(3):412–5.

18. Fattahi T, Steinberg B, Fernandes R, et al. Repair of nasal complex fractures the need for secondary septo-rhinoplasty. J Oral Maxillofac Surg 2006; 64(12):1785–9.

19. Borner U, Anschuetz L, Kaiser N, et al. Blunt nasal trauma in children: a frequent diagnostic challenge. Eur Arch Otorhinolaryngol 2019;276(1):85–91.

20. Cakabay T, Bezgin SU. Pediatric nasal traumas: contribution of epidemiological features to detect the distinction between nasal fractures and nasal soft tissue injuries. J Craniofac Surg 2018;29(5): 1334–7.

21. Chukwulebe S, Hogrefe C. The diagnosis and management of facial bone fractures. Emerg Med Clin North Am 2019;37(1):137–51.

22. Cohn JE, Othman S, Toscano M, et al. Nasal bone fractures: differences amongst sub-specialty consultants. Ann Otol Rhinol Laryngol 2020;129(11): 1120–8.

Approach to Orbital Fractures After Athletic Injuries

John Flynn, MD*

KEYWORDS

• Orbital trauma • Orbital fracture • Orbital blowout

KEY POINTS

- Athletic injuries can frequently involve the bony orbit. Evaluation should include a comprehensive history and ocular examination. Computed tomography imaging is the gold standard for diagnostic testing.
- Orbital fractures can occur in isolation or as combined fractures with multiple orbital walls and/or zygomaticomaxillary complex fractures. Depending on the fracture pattern, considerations for vision and intracranial complications must be considered.
- Management of orbital floor fractures can be broken down into 3 main treatment pathways: urgent surgical intervention, delayed surgical intervention, and nonoperative management. Most orbital fractures do not require urgent surgical intervention and repair can be completed within 2 weeks of the injury.
- The goal of operative management of orbital fractures includes restoration of globe position, mobility, and orbital volume. Intraoperative computed tomography has become more frequently used and can lead to improved intraoperative plate positioning.

INTRODUCTION

Orbital trauma is a commonly seen athletic injury. It is estimated that between 40,000 and 600,000 physician visits per year are sports-related ocular injuries in the United States.[1] Sports-related ocular injuries also have potential for major morbidity. Orbital trauma is the second leading cause of blindness and sports are responsible for one-third of eye injuries that lead to blindness.[2] Because of the risk of blindness, care for the globe is of utmost importance. Certain sports have a greater propensity for orbital injury and those include baseball/softball, paintball, basketball, racquetball, football, and soccer. Maxillofacial trauma makes up approximately 21% of sports-related fractures, and orbital floor fractures make up about 17% of that cohort.[3] With a high degree of concurrent cerebral and ocular injuries, care for the patient with ocular trauma must be appropriately triaged.[4] Once patients have undergone safe triage, care for orbital trauma can occur. Orbital fractures can range from small, nondisplaced fractures, to large fractures with significant orbital disruption. Owing to their complex nature, a large range of factors must be considered in the management of orbital trauma.

EVALUATION

Evaluation should begin with clinical history, comprehensive review of systems, and physical examination. In patients who sustain traumatic injury to the face, orbital trauma should be suspected. Maintaining a high index of suspicion can help enhance the detection of occult fractures. A complete ophthalmic evaluation should be performed. A focused history should include the

Department of Otolaryngology–Head and Neck Surgery, University of Kansas School of Medicine, The University of Kansas Medical Center, 3901 Rainbow Boulevard, MS 3010, Kansas City, KS 66160, USA
* Corresponding author. 8 Emerson Place #801 Boston MA 02114.
E-mail address: flynnjohnp@gmail.com

Facial Plast Surg Clin N Am 30 (2022) 31–45
https://doi.org/10.1016/j.fsc.2021.08.003
1064-7406/22/© 2021 Elsevier Inc. All rights reserved.

mechanism of injury and current symptoms. A prior history of ocular conditions and pathologies should also be performed. Visual acuity of individual eyes, pupillary response, and extraocular mobility are paramount to the initial examination. Although enophthalmos and hypoglobus are not always manifested in the acute setting, these findings are associated with increased intraorbital volume after large orbital fractures. Enophthalmos is best detected by taking exophthalmometry measurements (**Fig. 1**).[5]

Extraocular mobility limitations are common after orbital fracture, but several distinct etiologies can lead to this finding. Both orbital edema and hemorrhage involving the muscles may lead to restriction in movements. Entrapment of muscle or perimuscular tissue can also lead to restrictions, but this is usually associated with pain and guarding. An increase in intraocular pressure greater than 4 mm Hg when looking in the direction of the diplopia may also signify restriction. Contrarily, paralytic diplopia because of nerve injury will not demonstrate increased intraocular pressure or pain.[6] Multidirectional mobility limitations or "frozen globe," may signify retrobulbar hematoma. This typically manifests with concurrent increased intraocular pressure and proptosis. This is a medical emergency in which canthotomy and cantholysis should be performed to release pressure on the optic nerve.

Evaluation of the ocular adnexa should also be performed. The examination should include the lacrimal system, medial and lateral canthal tendons, and evaluation of telecanthus. A full cranial nerve examination should be performed to evaluate for trigeminal and facial nerve injury.

Ophthalmology consultation and evaluation for all patients with orbital trauma should be considered, as ophthalmologist may recognize ocular pathology at greater rates than nonophthalmologist.[7,8] A thorough ophthalmologic examination can help identify ocular foreign bodies, rupture of the globe, altered intraocular pressure, retinal and posterior segment pathology, and lens dislocation. Approximately, 20% of orbital fractures have some associated ocular pathology. The most common findings include commotio retinae, traumatic mydriasis, and traumatic iritis.[9]

ADDITIONAL TESTING

The mainstay of diagnostic testing after orbital trauma is radiological evaluation. Computed tomography (CT) imaging is the gold standard for evaluation of the bony orbit. Fine cuts (<2 mm) should be performed to achieve optimal evaluation of the orbital bone. CT imaging should be thoroughly evaluated in multiple planes. The coronal plane helps identify medial wall fractures as well as orbital floor fractures (**Fig. 2**).[10] Inferior entrapment may demonstrate a rounded or vertically oriented ovoid shape to the inferior rectus muscle. In addition, inferior rectus rounding may occur during disruption of the fascial sling which supports the orbit.[11] The sagittal plane can aid in understanding the depth and length of an orbital floor fracture.

MRI is generally not necessary in the assessment of orbital trauma. MRI should not be performed as first-line imaging. A CT or plain film should be acquired first to rule out foreign bodies within the orbit. Despite CT imaging being the mainstay of diagnostic testing, some have suggested that soft tissue intraorbital injury may play a larger role in predicting outcomes after orbital fracture. For this reason, MRI has been suggested as a means to help further define treatment strategies in difficult cases.[11] If there is concern for optic nerve, extraocular muscle, or cavernous sinus injury, then MRI may have additional utility.[6]

Numerous studies have analyzed fracture size, location (involvement of anterior or posterior walls, orbital strut), soft tissue displacement, inferior rectus rounding, and other features to predict the development of latent enophthalmos, but these have had varied success.[12–16] Orbital volume ratios have also been used to predict the need for surgical intervention with inconsistency.[16,17]

ORBITAL FRACTURE PATTERNS
Orbital Floor

The bony orbit is a conical structure and has a volume of approximately 30 mL.[18] The inferior orbital wall, or orbital floor, forms the roof of the maxillary sinus. It is formed by the maxillary, zygomatic, and palatine bones. The infraorbital nerve courses the length of the orbital floor. As the most dependent portion of the orbit, orbital contents including inferior rectus and orbital fat rest along the floor. Orbital floor fractures may or may not include the inferior orbital rim. Fractures of the orbital floor are the most common orbital fracture pattern. The floor is thinnest medial to the infraorbital nerve, and this serves as the most common location for fracture.[6]

Medial Orbital Wall

The medial orbital wall is the thinnest of all orbital walls. It is formed by the maxillary, ethmoid, lacrimal, and sphenoid bones. It is thinnest along the lamina papyracea of the ethmoid bone. The ethmoid bone joins with the orbital roof at the frontoethmoidal suture line. It is at this point where

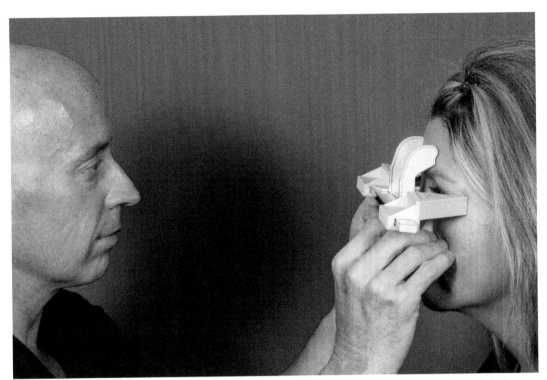

Fig. 1. The exophthalmometer is used to take objective measurements for determination of enophthalmos.

anterior and posterior ethmoid foramina are located. Their respective ethmoidal arteries course through these foramina after branching from the ophthalmic artery. The anterior ethmoid

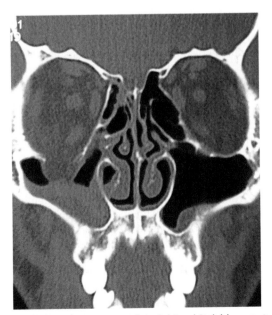

Fig. 2. The appearance of a right orbital blow out fracture on coronal cuts from computed tomography imaging.

neurovascular bundle is typically 20 to 25 mm posterior to the lacrimal crest, whereas the posterior ethmoid neurovascular bundle is another 12 mm posterior to the anterior foramina. The optic canal typically lies 4 to 8 mm posterior to the posterior foramina[6] (**Fig. 3**).[10] Medial wall fractures can occur in isolation or in combination with orbital floor fractures. Inferiorly, the medial orbital wall transitions to the thick orbital strut bone which is often resistant to fracture.[19]

Orbital Roof

The frontal bone and the lesser wing of the sphenoid make up the orbital roof. The roof separates the orbit from the frontal sinus as well as the anterior cranial fossa. Orbital roof fractures are less common, but their potential for morbidity is high. There are 4 general classifications for orbital roof fractures: "blow in fractures" with inferior displacement of the roof, "blow up fractures" with superior roof displacement into the anterior cranial fossa, supraorbital rim fractures, and frontal sinus fractures.[20] Fractures that involve the anterior cranial fossa may lead to pneumocephalus or a dural tear resulting in cerebrospinal fluid leak. A high-impact injury is required to sustain a roof fracture as there is protection from the surrounding frontal sinus. When orbital roof fractures occur,

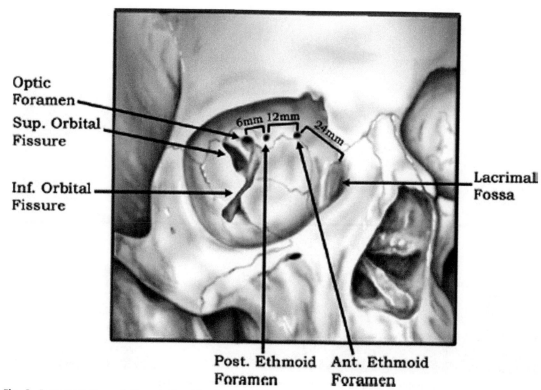

Fig. 3. Demonstration of the relationships between the anterior and posterior ethmoidal arteries and optic foramina as measured from the lacrimal crest.

concurrent traumatic brain injury with intracranial hemorrhage can be seen in approximately two-thirds of cases.[21] Evaluation of orbital roof fractures should involve not only the facial trauma team but also ophthalmology and neurosurgery.

Combined Orbital Fractures

Combined fractures of both the orbital floor and medial orbital wall are not uncommon and can occur in up to 35% of cases.[22] As the orbital wall(s) defect size is increased, the degree of enophthalmos is also increased. Patients with combined fractures have been shown to have a statistically significant change in exophthalmometric measurements compared to those with isolated orbital floor fracture.[22] These fracture patterns can make reconstruction challenging if there is a loss of inferonasal support at the orbital strut. In addition, involvement of the inferior oblique muscle near the lacrimal fossa can complicate reconstruction.

MANAGEMENT
Orbital Floor Fractures

Management of orbital floor fractures can be broken down into 3 main treatment pathways: urgent surgical intervention, delayed surgical intervention, and nonoperative management. Most orbital fractures do not require urgent surgical intervention and repair can be completed within 2 weeks of the injury.

Immediate repair (within the first 48 hours after injury) should be performed if there is a concern for oculocardiac reflex which manifests as bradycardia, nausea, and/or syncope. This reflex occurs secondary to soft tissue entrapment or increased intraorbital pressure. The ophthalmic division of the trigeminal nerve carries afferent fibers to the ciliary ganglion. Vagal nerve efferent signals are then transmitted to both the cardiac and gastric tissues.[23] Life-threatening cardiac arrhythmia may ensue if no intervention is performed. In the absence of oculocardiac reflex, immediate repair has remained controversial and management likely depends on training and experience.

Specific indications for orbital floor repair include clinical (positive force duction testing) and radiological concern for entrapment, enophthalmos greater than 2 mm, and orbital wall defects greater than 2 cm². If enophthalmos develops immediately after injury, then this will not improve without surgical repair. In addition, pediatric trapdoor (white-eye blowout) fractures in which orbital tissue is trapped between bony agments warrants urgent repair.[24] In cases of entrapment or incarceration, prolonged muscle ischemia can lead to a Volkmann's type contracture of the extraocular muscles.[25] Evidence of globe rupture, hyphema, or other ocular injuries should *delay* internal orbit repair approaches until an ophthalmology evaluation and repair has been completed.[5]

In cases that do not necessitate immediate repair, delayed surgical intervention can be considered. Repeat evaluation should be performed within 2 weeks of injury. A better clinical evaluation can be performed after orbital edema and hemorrhage have improved. Transient diplopia is a common finding in the immediate postinjury setting, and this may be due to muscle contusion and/or intraorbital edema. Edema typically improves within 2 weeks of injury, and any persistent diplopia is a compelling sign for intervention. Delayed repair affords improved exposure and mitigates risk of orbital compartment syndrome; however, delay does increase the risk of impinged tissue undergoing fibrosis and resulting in chronic diplopia.[26,27]

Indications for delayed repair of the orbital floor include latent enophthalmos, significant hypoglobus, and progressive hypesthesia along the infraorbital nerve.[24] Significant rounding of the inferior rectus muscle in which the height-to-width ratio is greater than 1.00 has been shown to be predictive of development of latent enophthalmos.[28] Difficult clinical decision-making occurs when ocular motility has improved, but enophthalmos persists. In these scenarios, fracture defect size on CT imaging and individualized patient approach can be helpful. Athletes likely have a lesser degree of tolerance for gaze-induced diplopia compared to an elderly, more sedentary patient.

In some cases, patients may present in a delayed fashion, months to years after injury. In these cases, it has been shown that delayed repair is still useful. Scawn and colleagues repaired 20 late presenting orbital floor fractures (mean presentation time of 19 months after injury) in patients with greater than 2 mm of enophthalmos or diplopia within 30° of primary gaze. Even at a later time of initial presentation, improvement in symptoms is still achievable.[29]

In patients with minimal diplopia (not in the primary or downward gaze fields), good ocular mobility, and no enophthalmos or hypoglobus, they are unlikely to require repair.[24] Additional management for nonoperative patients should include sinus precautions and education regarding avoidance of nose-blowing, as this can force air into the orbit. In severe cases, tension pneumo-

orbit can lead to a compartment syndrome resulting in optic nerve compression and blindness.[26] Cold compress and head of bed elevation can reduce orbital edema. If lagophthalmos is present, then corneal protection is required. Best evidence suggests that prophylactic antibiotic use is of minimal utility in upper or midface facial fractures.[30] There is some evidence that patients with pre-existing sinus disease or active sinus infection may be at increased risk of development of orbital cellulitis.[31]

Medial Orbital Wall Fractures

The clinical consequence of fractures along the medial orbital wall can be difficult to predict, but in general, these fractures can be managed conservatively. There is less data regarding clinical guidelines for repair of isolated medial wall fractures, but extrapolation of isolated orbital floor guidelines has led to recommendations. Entrapment based on positive forced duction testing of the medial rectus as well as early enophthalmos are indications for repair. The more common pathophysiologic mechanism by which medial wall fractures limit patient function is by change in orbital volume. Because of this, latent enophthalmos and diplopia also warrant repair.[32]

Orbital Roof Fractures

Recognition of orbital roof fractures is paramount in reducing intracranial or orbital complications. Most orbital roof fractures are minimally displaced and can be managed conservatively. There is a lack of consensus on exactly which symptoms warrant surgery versus conservative management. Because of the rarity of these fractures, guidelines are largely anecdotal, and treatment should be individualized.[20] Blow-in fractures that lead to exophthalmos, levator dysfunction, or entrapment should be considered for undergoing repair. Blow-up fractures that lead to dural tears, bone fragments in the anterior cranial fossa, and refractory oculorrhea should also be considered for repair.[20]

Concurrent Orbital and Zygomaticomaxillary Complex Fractures

It is not uncommon for both orbital and zygomaticomaxillary complex (ZMC) fractures to occur concurrently. This is most commonly seen when an inferior orbital fissure fracture line extends along the orbital floor toward the orbital process of the maxilla and infraorbital rim.[33] Traditionally, orbital floor exploration was part of the treatment paradigm for ZMC fractures. With the increased use of CT imaging, the rate of orbital exploration significantly dropped from 90% in 1985 to 30% in 1989.[34] But even with increased use of preoperative imaging, there is still a concern that during ZMC reduction a change in orbital volume could precipitate enophthalmos or diplopia. Ellis and colleagues looked at this issue and demonstrated that inferior displacement of the orbital floor is rare (6 of 65 cases), and when it occurs, the amount of displacement is small. Because of these findings, it is generally thought that approach and repair of small orbital fractures are not necessary after appropriate reduction of the ZMC. Intraoperative imaging can be used for assessment of orbital fractures following ZMC reduction, but this has been shown to result in a rare need to repair the orbit.[35] Despite the evidence supporting observation of small concurrent orbital fractures when repairing the ZMC, many still concurrently explore and/or repair the orbit in clinical practice.[36]

Management of Pediatric Orbital Trauma

Pediatric orbital fractures vary in their fracture pattern as the child ages due to the ongoing developmental anatomy. The immaturity of the pediatric skeleton demonstrates higher levels of cancellous bone which gives the pediatric facial bones higher levels of elasticity and resistance to fracture. This characteristically results in "greenstick" fractures. As the child ages, increased bone mineralization occurs, and the bone becomes more rigid. In addition, the pediatric population has a greater cranial:facial ratio. Because of the partial or absent pneumatization of the sinuses in younger pediatric populations, there is even greater resistance to fracture. In fact, it has been determined that before age 7 years, orbital roof fractures are more common than orbital floor fractures.[37]

Although periorbital edema and ecchymosis are commonly seen in adult patients with orbital fractures, pediatric patients may present without these findings. This type of fracture is called a "white eye" blowout fracture.[38] These fractures have a higher rate of entrapment when compared with adult patients because of the elasticity of the pediatric bone.[39] Assessment of entrapment may be more difficult in the pediatric patient, and as such, oculocardiac reflex or nausea and vomiting may be the most apparent clinical finding.[40]

Because of the resiliency of the pediatric elastic connective tissues and ligamentous attachments, they are less likely to develop enophthalmos and vertical dystopia. Pediatric fractures are typically able to be observed at higher incidence than adult fractures. Patients with minimal diplopia, unrestricted ocular motility, no evidence of muscle or soft tissue entrapment on CT imaging, and

improvement within 2 weeks can be observed. In cases of entrapment or enophthalmos, surgical intervention is warranted. Pediatric orbital fractures are typically approached similar to adults, but unlike adults, rigid titanium mesh may not be the ideal fixation material for the immature facial skeleton. Instead, resorbable plates have been suggested.[41]

Return to Play After Orbital Trauma in Athletes

There are no set guidelines for return to play after orbital trauma. Determination for return to play is largely based on the athlete's ability to function at his or her pretraumatized level. If binocular vision is restored and patient is without functional deficits, then consideration for play can be made. If an injury has occurred in a patient's only seeing eye, then great caution should be taken before considering return to play.

When considering return to play, athletes should be counseled on proper protective equipment. Evidence suggests that 90% of ocular injuries are preventable with proper eye protection. Sport-specific eyewear has been recommended by the American Academy of Pediatrics and the American Academy of Ophthalmology.[42] Regrettably, it is estimated that only 15% of children in organized sports adhere to proper eye protection guidelines.[2]

There has been a growing trend of professional athletes donning protective prosthetic face masks after maxillofacial trauma. This use has triggered interest among younger, nonprofessional athletes.[43] There is inherent risk to early return to play after orbital fracture, but prosthetic facemasks can provide some degree of protection against refracture. These facemasks are designed to redistribute forces acquired during sports-related contact to protect the maxillofacial skeleton. Over-the-counter facemasks are available as an affordable option, whereas custom-made masks can also be created from a mold of the player's face. Currently, there is little scientific evidence to suggest superiority of certain facemask types for prevention of repeat injury.

SURGICAL TECHNIQUES
Approaches to the Orbital Floor

Subcilliary/subtarsal approach
Both the subcilliary and subtarsal approaches are transcutaneous approaches, which were originally described in 1944.[44] Both these approaches begin with the placement of a temporary lateral tarsorrhaphy stitch, which can be used for eye protection and retraction. Incision for the subcilliary

approach is carried out 2 mm below the lash line and runs parallel to its course. The incision should not be carried more medially than the lower lid punctum but can extend 15 mm beyond the lateral canthus. Dissection is carried inferior to the tarsal plate in a plane superficial to the orbicularis oculi to maintain the lower lid structural support. The dissection then continues toward the orbital rim in a preseptal plane until the periosteum is encountered. At this point, the periosteum is incised, and periosteal elevator is used to expose the orbital floor (**Fig. 4**).[10] If a subtarsal approach is used, then the incision is created in the subtarsal fold (approximately 5–7 mm below the lash line). Dissection through the orbicularis oculi should be performed 2 to 3 mm below the level of the skin incision to decrease the likelihood of ectropion or scar inversion. Although these approaches provide excellent exposure to the orbital floor, they will typically have a visible scar and increased probability of lower lid malposition compared with the transconjunctival approach.[45]

Transconjunctival approach

The transconjunctival approach has largely supplanted the transcutaneous approaches because of its decreased risk of lower lid malpositioning. Lateral canthotomy and inferior cantholysis can also be performed to greatly enhance exposure. A Jaeger lid plate is used to retract and protect the globe. Eversion of the lower eyelid is then performed, and the incision is carried out using a Colorado tip dissector through the lower lid conjunctiva at least 2 mm below the tarsal plate. This approach can be subclassified as either preseptal or postseptal (**Fig. 5**).[46] If using the preseptal approach, then dissection continues deep to the orbicularis oculi, but superficial to the orbital septum. This is best accomplished bluntly with a cotton tip applicator. A suture (5–0 silk) can be placed through the conjunctival flap for upward retraction and globe protection. If a postseptal approach is used, then blunt dissection is carried out deep to the orbital septum. Orbital fat will be encountered but is contained by malleable retractor while the lower lid is retracted with a Ragnell. The periosteum of the inferior orbital rim can then be incised using a Colorado dissector. Elevation of the periosteum continues until desired exposure along the orbital floor is obtained. After adequate plating is performed, the conjunctival incision should be reapproximated, but does not require closure. The transconjunctival approach has advantage in that there is no external scar and less risk of ectropion compared to transcutaneous approaches. The orbital fat content can make the postseptal approach more challenging, but it affords less risk for postoperative lower lid malpositioning without violation between the orbicularis oculi and the orbital septum.

Transantral approach

This approach is ideally performed with endoscopic assistance. It begins with a gingivobuccal incision using electrocautery over the maxillary alveolus. Care should be taken to maintain an adequate cuff of tissue for closure on the gingival side. The maxillary periosteum is incised and elevated to the level of the infraorbital nerve. Once adequate exposure of the left maxillary sinus is achieved, an osteotome and Kerrison rongeur are used to perform an osteotomy along the anterior maxillary sinus wall. The defect is widened so that it can accommodate an endoscope and any needed instrumentation. Hopkin's rod nasal endoscopes, both 0° and 30° 4 mm scopes, can be used to visualize the orbital fracture. Any overlying mucosa is elevated, and the fracture can be reduced. This technique can be used as an adjunct to the standard approaches or as an isolated approach. After reduction and fixation are achieved, the gingivobuccal incision is closed. This approach affords excellent visibility of the posterior shelf, but there is difficulty in reconstruction lateral to the infraorbital nerve.[47]

Approach to the Medial Orbital Wall

Lynch approach

Access to most of the medial orbital wall can be achieved via this transcutaneous approach. Incision is carried out along the ipsilateral medial orbital rim. The incision beings at the inferior aspect of the medial brow and descends inferiorly to the superior aspect of the nasofacial junction. Dissection continues to the periosteum of the medial orbital rim using monopolar cautery. Care is taken to stay superior to the medial canthal attachments. A periosteal elevator is then used to elevate along the medial orbital wall. If the superomedial orbit is exposed, then identification and ligation of the ethmoidal arteries may be needed. After addressing the fracture, the skin incision should be closed. This approach can provide excellent exposure but is limited in use due to scarring and the possibility of medial canthal webbing.[48]

Transcaruncular approach

The approach has replaced the Lynch approach as the standard access method to the medial orbit. It begins with a 12 to 15 mm incision posterior to the caruncle, but anterior to the semilunar fold.[49] The upper and lower eyelids can be retracted with Demares or fine forceps. The incision can

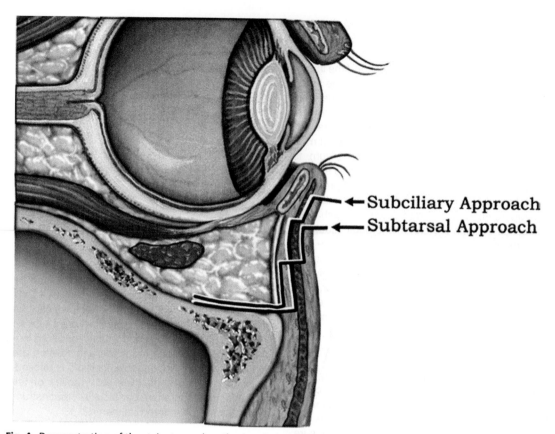

→ Subciliary Approach
→ Subtarsal Approach

Fig. 4. Demonstration of the stair-stepped method to the subcilliary and subtarsal approaches to the orbital floor.

be made through the body of the caruncle, which may serve as a landmark for closure (**Fig. 6**).[50] Initial dissection can be carried out with Stevens tenotomy scissors or monopolar cautery. Stevens tenotomy scissors should be used to palpate 1 to 2 mm posterior to the lacrimal crest and dissection should proceed toward the medial orbital wall. Care is taken to stay posterior to the lacrimal apparatus and Horner's muscle. The plane of dissection should proceed posterior to Horner's muscle, but medial to the medial orbital septum (**Fig. 7**).[50] If the orbital septum can be maintained, then this aids in containing the orbital fat. Once the periosteum is encountered, it should be widely incised using a Colorado dissector and elevated using a sharp elevator. The periosteum can be used as a membrane to help contain orbital fat. If the superomedial orbit is exposed, then identification and ligation of the ethmoidal arteries may be needed. After fracture repair, the incision can be closed with 6 to 0 fast gut suture in an interrupted fashion. Advantages of this approach include the avoidance of visible scars and medial canthal webbing.

When wide exposure to both the medial orbital wall and orbital floor are needed, this approach can be combined with a transconjunctival approach. When combining these approaches, the inferior oblique may need to be sharply divided near its origin. If this occurs, then a preplaced suture can be useful for reapproximation at the conclusion of the case. The inferior oblique should be released at its bony origin to avoid injury to the body of the muscle.

Transnasal approach

The transnasal approach is also an endoscopically assisted technique. It is usually combined with an orbitotomy approach such as the transcaruncular approach. The transnasal approach begins with intranasal decongestion. The 4 mm 0° nasal endoscope is introduced into the ipsilateral nasal cavity and the uncinate process is identified and uncinectomy is performed.[51] The natural ostium of the maxillary sinus can then be identified and widened following standard procedure for maxillary antrostomy. The ethmoid bulla should be identified and removed along with complete anterior ethmoidectomy. At this point, the lamina papyracea is identified. This bony plane can be followed until the medial orbital wall defect is identified. Orbital contents may become apparent at this

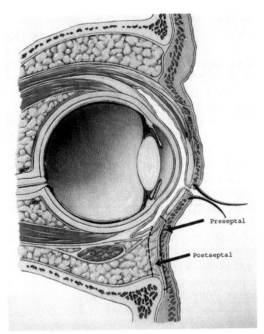

Fig. 5. Depiction of the preseptal and postseptal subclassification to the transconjunctival approach.

point and care should be taken to avoid further injury. These contents can then be reduced either transnasally or via orbitotomy. After adequate reduction, the orbital implant should be placed through the orbitotomy, but guided into correct position with endoscopic guidance and visualization.

Approaches to the Orbital Roof

Lateral brow approach
Exposure of the orbital roof, as well as the zygomaticofrantal and zygomaticosphenoid suture

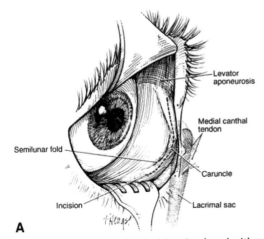

A

Fig. 6. The transcaruncular incision is placed either overlying the caruncle or just posterior to the caruncle, but anterior to the semilunar fold.

lines, can be accomplished with both the lateral brow and upper blepharoplasty approaches.[10] The lateral brow approach begins with a 2 to 3 cm incision just inferior to the hair follicles of the lateral eyebrow. This incision can be made within the brow but may lead to alopecia. Dissection is carried through the skin, subcutaneous tissue, and orbicularis oculi muscle. The periosteum is encountered and then incised. This is elevated with a periosteal elevator until the desired exposure is obtained. Closure should be performed by first reapproximating the periosteum. The orbicularis is reapproximated and sutured and the skin is then closed. Although this technique is advantageous because of its simplicity, it has largely been replaced by the upper blepharoplasty approach due to visible scarring and brow alopecia.

Upper blepharoplasty approach
The supratarsal crease is marked out and carried laterally within a skin fold beyond the lateral canthus as indicated based on the needed visualization (**Fig. 8**).[52] The skin is incised, and the orbicular oculi muscle is encountered. Fibers of this muscle should be incised parallel to their course. The dissection is carried superolaterally toward the orbital rim in a plane superficial to the orbital septum and lacrimal gland. Once the rim is encountered, the periosteum is incised and elevated using a periosteal elevator (**Fig. 9**).[10] Closure should be performed by first reapproximating the periosteum. The orbicularis is reapproximated and sutured and the skin is then closed. Because this approach is cosmetically favorable to the lateral brow approach, it is the preferred method.

Coronal approach
The coronal approach provides broad unparalleled visualization of the orbits, zygomatic arch, and nasal bones. The benefits of this approach must be weighed against the risks of forehead numbness, injury to the frontal branch of the facial nerve, and alopecia. This approach may be indicated if there is extensive craniofacial trauma or if calvarial bone graft is needed.

INTRAOPERATIVE IMAGING, COMPUTER-ASSISTED SURGERY, AND VIRTUAL SURGICAL PLANNING

Intraoperative assessment of adequate reduction and fixation has been shown to be a useful adjunct to operative management of midface fractures.[53] The goal of operative management of orbital fractures includes restoration of globe position, mobility, and orbital volume. Although radiologic imaging can be performed postoperatively, there

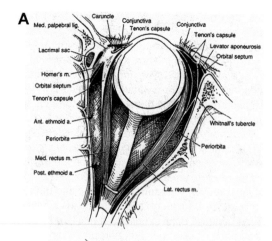

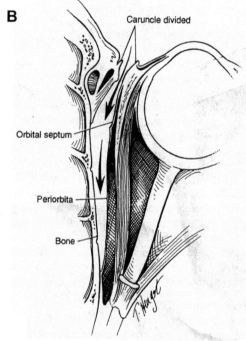

Fig. 7. The transcaruncular dissection is carried out posterior to the lacrimal apparatus and Horner's muscle (A). The periosteum of the medial orbital wall is identified and dissection within this plane occurs until the fracture is encountered (B).

is concern that suboptimal outcomes may go un-revised.[54] There are several adjuncts which can be used for intraoperative imaging including fluoroscopy, ultrasonography, spiral CT, and cone-beam CT (CBCT). As a relatively new technology, CBCT is not available everywhere, but its low cost, low radiation exposure, and overall utility have been demonstrated.[53] Cuddy and colleagues evaluated the use of intraoperative CT in facial trauma and found that an intraoperative revision was performed in 28% patients.[55] Of the anatomic

subsites, orbital revision had the highest rate of revision at 31% (**Fig. 10**).[56] The greater the complexity of the orbital repair, the greater the likelihood for intraoperative revision.[57] The use of this technology is time efficient and has been shown to add less than 15 minutes to the surgical procedure.[58]

Alternatively, intraoperative image guidance can be used for orbital reconstruction. The contralateral, untraumatized orbit can be mirrored onto the traumatized orbit to reconstruct its bony framework. This technique has been shown to be reliable and legitimate.[59] Bly and colleagues performed preoperative mirror image overlay with endoscopically assisted surgical navigation. This study used the navigation to confirm plate positioning, and demonstrated improved postoperative diplopia, orbital volume, and decreased need for revision surgery.[60] For more complex orbital defects, computer-assisted surgery can be used with virtual surgical planning and 3D-printed custom implants.[61,62]

Recent advances in machine learning and image recognition have been used in radiologic analyses. Several studies have demonstrated the ability of machine learning algorithms to predict fractures. This same technology has been used to automatically detect orbital fractures. This technology is still in its infancy but will likely become more prevalent. Future studies could use machine learning technology to help predict the need for surgical repair of fractures and assess postoperative outcomes.[63]

IMPLANT MATERIALS

Implant materials can broadly be divided into the following 4 main groups: alloplasts, allografts, autografts, and xenografts.[64] In regard to orbital implants, alloplasts (inert foreign materials that can be used for reconstruction) are most commonly used. Despite this, autografts (materials that have been moved from one area of the body to another) have been the historical gold standard.

The historical gold standard for orbital reconstruction has been autologous bone which is typically harvested from the calvarium.[64] This material has excellent biocompatibility but can be challenging when contouring for the orbit. Although the material is inexpensive, it does require a separate donor site with added surgical morbidity. Homologous bone has also been used as an allographic material, but because of its higher resorption rates, it is infrequently used.

Autologous cartilage can be used as a graft material and is typically harvested from the ear. It has many of the same biocompatibility advantages as

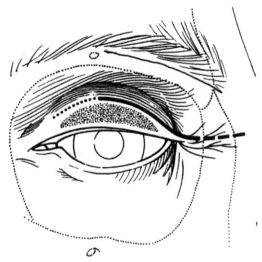

Fig. 8. The brow incision can be placed just inferior to the hair follicles to avoid alopecia. The upper blepharoplasty incision is placed within the supratarsal crease. This can be carried laterally within a crease along the lateral canthus.

autogenous bone; however, it is also not easily countered for the orbit. It has a lesser degree of structural support, inherent memory with unpredictable resorption.[64] Homologous cartilage has not been widely reported for internal orbit reconstruction in the literature. Because of the limited abilities of orbital reconstruction with autologous

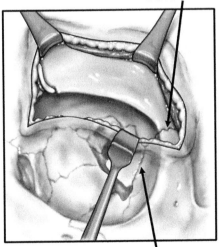

Zygomaticofrontal Suture

Zygomaticosphenoid Suture

Fig. 9. Demonstration of the zygomaticofrontal and zygomaticosphenoid sutures using the upper blepharoplasty approach.

and homologous grafting materials, alloplastic materials have become much more commonplace.[56]

Titanium Mesh Sheeting is frequently used in orbital reconstruction because of its favorable biocompatibility, structural stability, and ease of contouring and trimming to fit various orbital defects. The material is radiopaque and easily sterilized. As with all alloplasts, there is no donor site morbidity, but does come at an added cost. Plain sheets can be obtained for cutting by the surgeon or preformed orbital implants can be used. Custom patient-specific implants can also be created for complex defects.

Porous polyethylene is a controlled pore size polymer with high biocompatibility. Vascular ingrowth limits capsule formation and helps limit the host immune response. It also has good structural stability and ease of handling. It can be ordered as sheets, preformed orbital implants, or custom implants. Its main disadvantage is that it is not radiopaque; therefore, it is not visualized on intraoperative or postoperative imaging. Titanium-reinforced porous polyethylene combines the advantageous properties of both alloplastic materials. The titanium reinforcement allows for decreased shearing of the implant when screws are placed. It also becomes radiopaque, which aids in the analysis of implant positioning (**Fig. 11**).[56]

Resorbable sheeting (polylactide, polyglactin, and polydioxanone) fixation systems have become available and gained acceptance. As with other alloplasts, they are biocompatible and easily handled. These implants are not radiopaque. Their main advantage is their ability to resorb over time. In theory, this limits the possibility of lifelong side effects. The resorption of these implants occurs with hydrolysis and can result in a sterile inflammatory reaction.[65] Because of their resorption, these implants are likely not useful for large, complex orbital defects.

POSTOPERATIVE CARE

After any bony manipulation or implant placement, forced duction should be performed before completion of the procedure. While in the recovery room, patient should undergo visual acuity assessment as well as ocular motility testing. Overnight observation with light perception vision checks every 4 hours should be performed. Color discrimination is very sensitive for the detection of optic nerve injury.[5] Progressively worsening pain, changes in vision, or proptosis should raise concern for expanding retrobulbar hematoma. Head of bed elevation and cold compress will limit

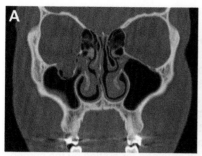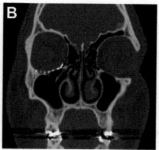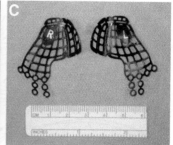

Fig. 10. (*A*) Preoperative CT image of orbital floor fracture. (*B*) Postoperative CT imaging demonstrating repair of orbital floor fracture. (*C*) Preformed titanium orbital floor implants.

orbital edema. Ophthalmic ointments will aid in moisturization of the cornea. Avoidance of nose blowing as well as strenuous activity and heavy lifting restrictions should be recommended for 2 weeks after surgery.

COMPLICATIONS

Diplopia is one of the most common complications after repair of orbital fractures. If diplopia is noted preoperatively, then it is possible to have some degree of postoperative diplopia after surgery related to edema.[5] Before concluding an orbital fracture repair, forced duction should be performed to ensure no entrapment is present. Intraoperative or postoperative imaging can also help confirm the resolution of entrapped tissue. If entrapped tissue was present before surgical intervention, then recovery of function may be prolonged or incomplete. This may result in persistent diplopia at which point ophthalmology consultation is recommended.

Vision loss after orbital surgery may indicate injury to the optic nerve or its vascular supply. The development of mydriasis intraoperatively is a sign that excessive pressure has been applied to the ocular contents. Vision loss can occur secondary to retrobulbar hemorrhage in the postoperative state. If vision changes, decreased color discrimination and/or increased ocular pressure occur, then canthotomy with cantholysis must be performed immediately at the bedside.[5] This should be followed by wound exploration and urgent ophthalmology consultation.

Lid malpositioning, as previously discussed, has a greater propensity to occur following transcutaneous approaches compared with transconjunctival approaches. There is an increased risk of entropion with using the preseptal transconjunctival approach secondary to scarring between the orbital septum and orbicularis oculi.[5] Any lid malpositioning in the acute postoperative state may be managed with observation and lid massage. Surgical repair of the lid may be required in persistently malpositioned cases.

CLINICS CARE POINTS

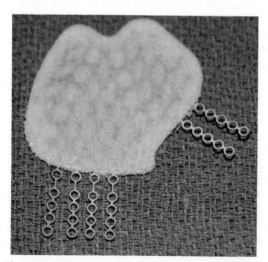

Fig. 11. Titanium-reinforced porous polyethylene orbital implant.

- Urgent surgical intervention for orbital floor fractures should occur after "white eye" trapdoor fractures or if oculocardiac response occurs.

- Indications for orbital floor repair include clinical and radiological concern for entrapment, enophthalmos greater than 2 mm, and orbital wall defects greater than 2 cm². In cases of entrapment or incarceration, prolonged muscle ischemia can lead to a Volkmann's type contracture of the extraocular muscles. Evidence of globe rupture, hyphema, or other ocular injury should *delay* internal orbit repair approaches until an ophthalmology evaluation.

- The transconjunctival approaches to the orbital floor have largely replaced the transcutaneous approaches. Similarly, the transcaruncular approach has largely replaced the Lynch approach to the medial orbital wall.

- Intraoperative computed tomography has become more frequently used and can lead to increased identification of plate malpositioning intraoperatively. This technology has been shown to be efficient and useful in challenging cases.

- There is a wide variety in orbital implant materials, but both titanium mesh sheeting and porous polyethylene are frequently used given their structural stability and ease of contouring.

- Although complications are rare, vision changes, loss of color discrimination, increasing ocular pressure, and pain are signs of retrobulbar hematoma. This should be treated emergently with canthotomy and inferior cantholysis.

DISCLOSURE

The author has nothing to disclose.

REFERENCES

1. Goldstein MH, Wee D. Sports injuries: an ounce of prevention and a pound of cure. Eye Cont Lens 2011;37:160–3.
2. Cass S. Ocular Injuries in Sports. Curr Sports Med Rep 2012;11(1):11–5.
3. Antoun JS, Lee KH. Sports-related maxillofacial fractures over an 11-year period. J Oral Maxillofac Surg 2008;66(3):504–8.
4. Ellis. Orbital trauma. Oral Maxillofac Surg Clin North Am 2012;24:629–48.
5. Humphrey CD, Kriet JD. Orbital fractures. In: Johnson JT, Rosen CA, editors. Bailey's head & neck surgery otolaryngology. 5th edition. Philadelphia: Wolters Kluwer/Lippincott Williams & Wilkins; 2014. p. 1225–40.
6. Timoney P, Tomasko K, Nunery WR. General principles of management of oribtal fractures. In: Servat JJ, Black EH, Nesi FA et al, editors. Smith and Nesi's ophthalmic plastic and reconstructive surgery. 4th edition. Springer. p. 1231–5.
7. Jabaley ME, Lerman M, Sanders HJ. Ocular injuries in orbital fractures. Plast Reconstr Surg 1975;56:410–4.
8. Cook T. Ocular and periocular injuries from orbital fractures. J Am Coll Surg 2002;195:831–4.
9. He D, Blomquist PH, Ellis E. Association between ocular injuries and internal orbital fractures. J Oral Maxillofac Surg 2007;65:713–20.
10. Humphrey CD, Kriet JD. Surgical approaches to the orbit. Oper Tech Otolayngol 2008;19:132–9.
11. Zimmer RM, Gellrich NC, Bulow SV, et al. Is there more to the clinical outcome in posttraumatic reconstruction of the inferior and medial orbital walls than accuracy of implant placement and implant surface contouring? A prospective multicenter study to identify predictors of clinical outcome. J Craniomaxillofac Surg 2018;46:578–87.
12. Hawes MJ, Dortzbach RK. Surgery on orbital floor fractures. Influence of time of repair and fracture size. Ophthalmology 1983;90(9):1066–70.
13. Harris GJ, Garcia GH, Logani SC, et al. Orbital blowout fractures: correlation of preoperative computed tomography and postoperative ocular motility. Trans Am Ophthalmol Soc 1998;96:329–47.
14. Higashino T, Hirabayashi S, Eguchi T, et al. Straightforward factors for predicting the prognosis of blow-out fractures. J Craniofac Surg 2011;22(4):1210–4.
15. Schouman T, Courvoisier DS, Van Issum C, et al. Can systematic computed tomographic scan assessment predict treatment decision in pure orbital floor blowout fractures? J Oral Maxillofac Surg 2012;70(7):1627–32.
16. Goggin J, Jupiter DC, Czerwinski M. Simple computed tomography-based calculations of orbital floor fracture defect size are not sufficiently accurate for clinical use. J Oral Maxillofac Surg 2015;73(1):112–6.
17. Choi SH, Kang DH, Gu JH. The correlation between the orbital volume ratio and enophthalmos in unoperated blowout fractures. Arch Plast Surg 2016;43(6):518–22.
18. Timoney P., Tomasko K., Nunery W.R. General principles of management of oribtal fractures. In: Servat J.J., Black E.H., Nesi F.A. et al, editors. Smith and Nesi's ophthalmic plastic and reconstructive surgery. 4th edition. Switzerland: Springer. p. 46.
19. Grob S, Yonkers M, Tao J. Orbital Fractures Repair. Semin Plast Surg 2017;31(1):31–9.
20. Lucas JP, Allen M, Nguyen BK, et al. Orbital roof fractures: an evidence-based approach. Facial Plast Surg Aesthet Med 2020;22(6):471–80.
21. Crossman JP, Morrison CD, Taylor HO, et al. Traumatic orbital roof fractures: interdisciplinary evaluation and management. Plast Reconstr Surg 2014;133(3):335–43.
22. Ordon AJ, Kozakiewicz M, Wilczynski M, et al. The influence of concomitant medial wall fracture on the results of orbital floor reconstruction. J Craniomaxillofac Surg 2018;46(4):573–7.

23. Shokri T, Alford M, Hammons M, et al. Management of orbital floor fractures. Facial Plast Surg 2019; 35(6):633–9.

24. Burnstine MA. Clinical recommendations for repair of isolated orbital floor fractures: an evidence-based analysis. Ophthalmology 2002;109(7):1207–10.

25. Sires BS, Stanley RB Jr, Levine LM. Oculocardiac reflex caused by orbital floor trapdoor fracture: an indication for urgent repair. Arch Ophthalmol 1998; 116(7):955–6.

26. Boyette JR, Pemberton JD, Bonilla-Velez JB. Management of orbital fractures: challenges and solutions. Clin Ophthalmol 2015;9:2127–37.

27. Brucoli M, Arcuri F, Cavenaghi R, et al. Analysis of complications after surgical repair of orbital fractures. J Craniofac Surg 2011;22:1387–90.

28. Malic DB, Tse R, Banerjee A, et al. Rounding of the inferior rectus muscle as a predictor of enophthalmos in orbital floor fractures. J Craniofac Surg 2007;18(1):127–32.

29. Scawn R, Lim L, Whipple K, et al. Outcomes of orbital blow-out fracture repair performed beyond 6 weeks after injury. Ophthal Plast Reconstr Surg 2016;32:296–301.

30. Mundinger GS, Borsuk DE, Okhah Z, et al. Antibiotics and facial fractures: evidence-based recommendations compared with experience-based practice. Craniomaxillofac Trauma Reconstr 2015; 8(1):64–78.

31. Ben Simon GJ, Bush S, Selva D, et al. Orbital cellulitis: a rare complication after orbital blowout fracture. Ophthalmology 2005;112(11):2030–4.

32. Choi M, Flores RL. Medial orbital wall fractures and the transcaruncular approach. J Craniofac Surg 2012;23:696–701.

33. Ellis E, Reddy L. Status of the internal orbit after reduction of zygomaticomaxillary complex fractures. J Oral Maxillofac Surg 2004;62:275–83.

34. Covington DS, Wainwright DJ, Teichgraeber JF, et al. Changing patterns in the epidemiology and treatment of zygoma fractures: 10-year review. J Trauma 1994;37:243.

35. Wilde F, Lorenz K, Ebner AK, et al. Intraoperative imaging with a 3D C-arm system after zygomatico-orbital complex fracture reduction. J Oral Maxillofac Surg 2013;71(5):894–910.

36. Flynn J, Lu GN, Kriet JD, et al. Trends in concurrent orbital floor repair during zygomaticomaxillary complex fracture repair. JAMA Facial Plast Surg 2019; 21(4):341–3.

37. Koltai PJ, Amjad I, Meyer D. Orbital fractures in children. Arch Otolaryngol Head Neck Surg 1995;121: 1375–9.

38. Jordan DR, Allen LH, White J, et al. Intervention within days for some orbital floor fractures: the white-eyed blowout. Ophthal Plast Reconstr Surg 1998;14:379–90.

39. Kwon JH, Moon JH, Kwon MS, et al. The differences of blowout fracture of the inferior orbital wall between children and adults. Arch Otolaryngol Head Neck Surg 2005;131:723–7.

40. Oppenheimer A, Monson L, Buchamn S. Pediatric orbital fractures. Craniomaxillofac Trauma Reconstr 2013;6:9–20.

41. Eppley BL. Use of resorbable plates and screws in pediatric facial fractures. J Oral Maxillofac Surg 2005;63:285–91.

42. American Academy of Pediatrics, Committee on Sports Medicine and Fitness, American Academy of Ophthalmology, Eye Health and Public Information Task Force. Protective eyewear for young athletes. Ophthalmology 2004;111:600–3.

43. Grandy JR, Fossett L, Wong BJF. Facemasks and basketball: NCAA division I consumer trends and a review of over-the-counter facemask. Laryngoscope 2016;126(5):1054–60.

44. Converse J. Two plastic operations for repair of orbit following severe trauma and extensive comminuted fracture. Arch Ophthalmol 1944;31(4):323–5.

45. Appling WD, Patrinely JR, Salzer TA. Transconjunctival approach vs subcilliary skin-muscle flap approach for orbital fracture repair. Arch Otolaryngol Head Neck Surg 1993;119:1000–7.

46. Ellis E, Zide MF. Transconjunctival approaches. In: Ellis E, Zide MF, editors. Surgical approaches to the facial skeleton. 2nd edition. Switzerland: Wolters Kluwer/Lippincott Williams & Wilkins; 2006. p. 41–64.

47. Farwell DG, Strong EB. Endoscopic repair of orbital floor fractures. Facial Plast Surg Clin North Am 2006; 14:11–6.

48. Lynch RC. The technique of a radical frontal sinus operation which has given me the best results. Laryngoscope 1921;31(1):1–5.

49. Goldberg RA, Mancini R, Demer JL, et al. The transcaruncular approach: surgical anatomy and technique. Arch Facial Plast Surg 2007;9(6):443–7.

50. Shorr N, Baylis HI, Goldberg RA, et al. Transcaruncular approach to the medial orbit and orbital apex. Ophthalmology 2000;107(8):1459–63.

51. Rhee JS, Chen CT. Endoscopic approach to medial orbital wall fractures. Facial Plast Surg Clin North Am 2006;14:17–23.

52. Kung DS, Kaban LB. Supratarsal fold incision for approach to the superior lateral orbit. Oral Surg Oral Med Oral Pathol Oral Radiol Endod 1996; 81(5):522–5.

53. Van Hout WMMT, Van Cann EM, Muradin MSM, et al. Intraoperative Imaging for the repair of zygomaticomaxillary fractures: a comprehensive review of the literature. J Craniomaxillofac Surg 2014;42(8): 1918–23.

54. van den Bergh B, Goey Y, Forouzanfar T, et al. Postoperative radiographs after maxillofacial trauma:

sense or nonsense? Int J Oral Maxillofac Surg 2011; 40:1373–6.

55. Cuddy K, Khatib B, Bell RB, et al. Use of intraoperative computed tomography in craniomaxillofacial trauma surgery. J Oral Maxillofac Surg 2018;76(5): 1016–25.

56. Potter JK, Malmquist M, Ellis E. Biomaterials for reconstruction of the internal orbit. Oral Maxillofac Surg Clin North Am 2012;24(4):609–27.

57. Shyu V, Chen HH, Chen CH, et al. Clinical outcome following intraoperative computed tomography- assisted secondary orbital reconstruction. J Plast Reconstr Aesthet Surg 2021;74(2):341–9.

58. Shaye DA, Tollefson TT, Strong EB. Use of intraoperative computed tomography for maxillofacial reconstructive surgery. JAMA Facial Plast Surg 2015; 17(2):113–9.

59. Jansen J, Dubois L, Schreus R, et al. Should virtual mirroring be used in the preoperative planning of an orbital reconstruction? J Oral Maxillofac Surg 2018; 76:380–7.

60. Bly RA, Chang SH, Cudejkova M, et al. Computer-guided orbital reconstruction to improve outcomes. JAMA Facial Plast Surg 2013;15(2):113–20.

61. Scolozzi P. Applications of 3D orbital computer-assisted surgery (CAS). J Stomatol Oral Maxillofac Surg 2017;118(4):217–23.

62. Day KM, Phillips PM, Sargent LA. Correction of a posttraumatic orbital deformity using three-dimensional modeling, virtual surgical planning with computer-assisted design, and three-dimensional printing of custom implants. Craniomaxillofac Trauma Reconstr 2018;11(1):78–82.

63. Li L, Song X, Guo Y, et al. Deep convolutional neural networks for automatic detection of orbital blowout fractures. J Craniofac Surg 2020;31:400–3.

64. Strong B. Orbital fractures: pathophysiology and implant materials for orbital reconstruction. Facial Plast Surg 2014;30:509–17.

65. Rubin JP, Yaremchuk MJ. Complications and toxicities of implantable biomaterials used in facial reconstructive and aesthetic surgery: a comprehensive review of the literature. Plast Reconstr Surg 1997; 100(5):1336–53.

Zygomaticomaxillary Fractures

Christine M. Jones, MD[a], Cecelia E. Schmalbach, MD, MSc[b],*

KEYWORDS

- Zygomaticomaxillary complex • Zygomatic arch • Orbitozygomatic fracture • Malar eminence
- Facial trauma • Facial fracture

KEY POINTS

- The zygomaticomaxillary complex (ZMC) is a tetrapod structure, with articulations at the zygomaticofrontal buttress, zygomaticomaxillary buttress, infraorbital rim, zygomatic arch, and zygomaticosphenoid suture.
- Displaced zygomaticomaxillary fractures cause midfacial flattening and widening.
- The zygomatic arch is difficult to visualize directly, and ZMC fractures are often treated with open reduction via minimal access incisions.
- The decision to perform one-, two-, three-, or four-point fixation of the zygomaticomaxillary complex depends on individual fracture characteristics.
- Reduction of the zygomatic bone to the greater wing of the sphenoid should be checked in all but single-point approaches, because it provides the most sensitive evaluation of three-dimensional reduction of the ZMC with the skull base.

INTRODUCTION

Fractures of the zygomaticomaxillary complex (ZMC) are common injuries, representing up to 25% of facial fractures.[1] In athletes, ZMC fractures can result from low- or high-velocity midfacial trauma.[2] Helmets have reduced the incidence of injury, but ZMC fracture is still common in baseball, basketball, and sports with a predisposition to falls from moderate heights, such as horseback riding,[3,4] among others.

The midface undergoes a substantial increase in size and ossification during the adolescent growth phase.[5] Children have a greater cranial-to-facial proportion, more flexible skeletal suture lines, unerupted dentition, and thicker overlying soft tissue, making midfacial fractures less common in young athletes than in late adolescents and adults (**Fig. 1**).[5–7] Fractures of the zygoma are about 70%

less common in pediatric patients than in adults,[5] and are uncommon before development of the globe pneumatization of the maxillary sinus is complete, about age 7.[8] The mechanism of injury, advances in protective equipment, and the age of typical athletes make ZMC fractures less common in athletes than in the general population, accounting for 4% to 8% of facial fractures sustained in sports.[3,4,9]

ANATOMY

The zygoma is a tetrapod cornerstone of the midface, representing the intersection of vertical, transverse, and sagittal facial buttresses (**Fig. 2**). The ZMC can fracture at any of these five articulations.

Fracture of the ZMC requires less force than most surrounding bones (**Fig. 3**).[10] The zygoma tends to become impacted, medially rotated, and

[a] Division of Plastic and Reconstructive Surgery, Lewis Katz School of Medicine at Temple University, 3401 North Broad Street, 4th Floor Parkinson Pavilion, Philadelphia, PA 19140, USA; [b] David Myers, MD Professor and Chair, Department of Otolaryngology – Head and Neck Surgery, Lewis Katz School of Medicine at Temple University, 3440 North Broad Street, Kresge West # 309, Philadelphia, PA 19140, USA
* Corresponding author.
E-mail address: Cecelia.Schmalbach@tuhs.temple.edu
Twitter: @CMJones_MD (C.M.J.)

Facial Plast Surg Clin N Am 30 (2022) 47–61
https://doi.org/10.1016/j.fsc.2021.08.004
1064-7406/22/© 2021 Elsevier Inc. All rights reserved.

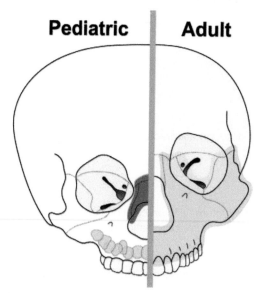

Pediatric   Adult

Fig. 1. Comparison of fracture locations significantly more frequent in pediatric (*left*, nasal fractures [*red*]) and adult (*right*, maxillary and zygomatic fractures [*blue*]) patients. Craniofacial skeletons are depicted at the same size to emphasize the small facial-to-cranial proportions in pediatric patients. (*From* Fujisawa K, Suzuki A, Yamakawa T, Onishi F, Minabe T. Pediatric-specific midfacial fracture patterns and management: Pediatric vs adult patients. J Craniofac Surg. 2020;31:e312-e315; with permission)

inferiorly displaced, which leads to widening and flattening of the midface.[11,12]

Isolated fractures of the zygomatic arch should be distinguished from those of the ZMC. The zygomatic arch typically bows inward, which may create a palpable or visible depression under the thin skin of the lateral midface.

The muscles of mastication pass from the temporal fossa and zygomatic arch to insert onto the

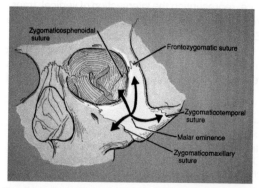

Fig. 2. Tetrapod structure of the ZMC. (*From* Strong EB, Gary C. Management of zygomaticomaxillary complex fractures. Fac Plast Surg Clin N Am. 2017;25:547–562; with permission)

mandible. Depressed fractures of the zygomatic arch or ZMC can cause trismus through impingement of the arch on the coronoid process of the mandible, adhesions between the arch and coronoid process, or direct injury to the muscles of mastication.[12,13]

The superomedial portion of the zygoma creates the lateral 40% of the orbital floor. This portion of the zygoma is thin and prone to buckling with an anterior or lateral impact.[14] For this reason, many ZMC fractures are accompanied by fractures of the orbital floor.

EVALUATION
History

A complete medical history should be obtained, focusing on mechanism of trauma, comorbidities, and symptoms (**Table 1**). High-energy athletic injuries, loss of consciousness, or the presence of spinal pain or peripheral neurologic symptoms necessitate a full trauma work-up. In children, zygomatic and orbital fractures have a higher likelihood of accompanying cervical spine injury.[15,16] Baseline visual changes should be identified. Recent use of nonsteroidal anti-inflammatory agents or anticoagulants may warrant discussion of the risk of perioperative bleeding.[17,18]

Physical Examination

A more accurate assessment is conducted after edema subsides, about 5 to 7 days post-trauma. Malar retrusion accompanies most operative fractures.[12] Step-offs may be palpable or visible along the buttresses. Pseudoptosis, vertical dystopia, inferior displacement of the lateral canthus, or increased scleral show may be more subtle signs of displacement.

Infraorbital hypoesthesia is often present, extending onto the upper lip and dentate maxilla. Trismus can represent an operative indication; approximately 4.5 cm of interincisal opening is necessary for full function. Subjective malocclusion may occur secondary to altered sensation in the region of the maxillary premolars and molars.

Signs of orbital trauma should be evaluated (see **Table 1**). Subconjunctival hemorrhage is a sensitive indicator of orbital fracture.[12,19,20] With concomitant orbital floor fractures, emergencies, such as entrapment, superior orbital fissure syndrome, orbital apex syndrome, and retrobulbar hematoma, must be ruled out. Concomitant major ocular or blinding injuries may be present in about 10% of patients; thus, consideration should be given for ophthalmologic evaluation in all ZMC fractures.[19,20]

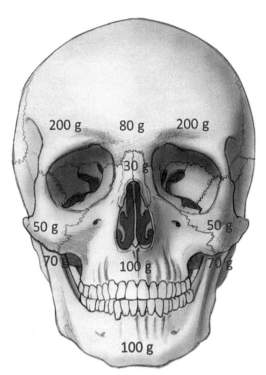

Fig. 3. Forces needed to fracture the facial bones. (*From* Viozzi CF. Maxillofacial and mandibular fractures in sports. Clin Sports Med. 2017;36:355–368; used with permission of Mayo Foundation for Medical Education and Research, all rights reserved)

Radiographic Evaluation

Maxillofacial computed tomography (CT) with thin cuts (0.625–1.0 mm) is the gold standard in evaluating for zygomaticomaxillary fractures.[21,22] In children, low-dose radiation protocols can limit exposure to ionizing radiation. Fracture lines and displacement are evaluated. On axial imaging, alignment of the zygomaticosphenoid buttress, infraorbital rim, and zygomatic arch is assessed

(Fig. 4). The zygomaticosphenoid buttress provides sagittal and transverse support to the zygoma and is a sensitive indicator of fracture displacement.[23,24] Retropositioning of the malar eminence is assessed on axial and three-dimensional imaging. Coronal and sagittal imaging are best to examine fractures and displacement of the zygomaticofrontal and zygomaticomaxillary buttresses. The degree of comminution should be noted, because this influences the number of points of fixation needed.

OPERATIVE MANAGEMENT
Virtual Surgical Planning

Preoperative virtual surgical planning (VSP) allows identification and reduction of individual fracture segments. Reduction is based on a mirror image of the uninjured contralateral side. In bilateral injuries or baseline deformity, a representative normative scan matched to the age and gender of the patient is used. Stereolithographic models are three-dimensional printed, modeling the fractured skeleton for better conceptualization, or simulating the reduced ZMC to prebend osteosynthesis plates.[25] Custom implants are fabricated to guide the proper skeletal reduction. VSP session data are combined with intraoperative navigation to compare the preoperative plan with operative execution.[1,26,27]

Timing and expense are barriers to widespread adoption. Commercial fabrication of custom-printed osteosynthesis plates currently takes approximately 2 weeks from the time of CT data submission. For acute trauma, timing is often not prompt enough to make VSP application practical, particularly for all but the most complex zygomaticomaxillary cases. With technologic advances and institutional sourcing, VSP may be more commonly used in the future.

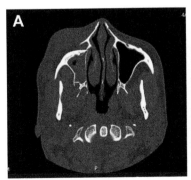
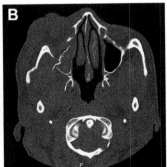
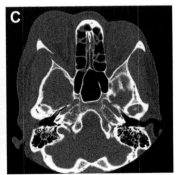

Fig. 4. Right ZMC fracture with displacement at infraorbital rim (*A*), zygomatic arch (*B*), and zygomaticosphenoid suture (*C*).

Table 1
Possible clinical signs and symptoms accompanying ZMC fractures.

Skeletal deformities	Ocular/ophthalmic symptoms	Sensory impairment	Oral symptoms	Nasal symptoms

• Asymmetry of the midface
• Depression/flattening of the malar prominence
• Flattening, hollowing (bony indentation) or broadening over the zygomatic arch
• Palpable step offs or gap deformities (infraorbital/lateral)
	• Periorbital edema or hematoma ("monocle hematoma")
	• Pseudoptosis
	• Increased scleral show
	• Downward slant of palpebral fissure or horizontal lid axis respectively
	• Malposition of the lateral canthus
	• Vertical shortening of the lower eyelid (ectropion)
	• Subconjunctival ecchymosis (temporal/medial)
	• Chemosis
	• Pupillary or globe level disparity (hypoglobus)
	• Proptosis bulbi
	• Enophthalmos (outward displacement of zygoma)
	• Exophthalmos (inward displacement of zygoma)
	• Subcutaneous periorbital air emphysema (skin crepitation)
		Sensory deficit (hypoesthesia, anesthesia) in the distribution of the following nerves:
		• Infraorbital nerve:
		  ○ lower eyelid
		  ○ upper lip
		  ○ ala and lateral sidewall of the nose
		• Zygomatiofacial nerve:
		  ○ malar eminence
		  ○ cheek
		• Zygomatiofacial nerve:
		  ○ lower lateral orbital rim
		  ○ anterior temporal/lateral/frontal region
			• Ecchymosis of the gingivobuccal maxillary sulcus
			• Subjective occlusal disorder due to altered sensation of the maxillary premolars/molars and gingiva, no objective malocclusion
			• Palpable contour disturbance of zygomaticomaxillaiy buttress
			• Restriction of mandibular opening (trismus) or closing—blockage of temporal muscle or coronoid process either by impacted zygomatic arch or retrodis-placed zygoma
				• Ipsilateral epistaxis
				• Ipsilateral hematosinus

- Pneumoexophthalmos
- Diplopia (neurogenic ocular motility disorder — III, IV, VI; enophthalmos; entrapment, revealed by forced duction test)
- Amaurosis
- Superior orbital fissure syndrome

From Cornelius CP. Zygomaticomaxillary complex fractures, zygomatic arch fractures. In: Principles of Internal Fixation of the Craniomaxillofacial Skeleton – Trauma and Orthognathic Surgery. Thieme;2012:205–221; with permission. Copyright AO Foundation, Switzerland.

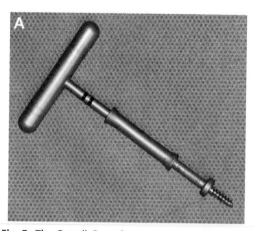 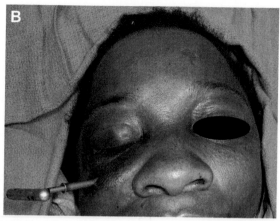

Fig. 5. The Carroll-Gerard screw is a threaded tool (*A*) that is placed through the lower eyelid incision or percutaneously (*B*) to assist with reduction or stabilize the ZMC during osteosynthesis.

Timing

Allowing time for facial edema to subside improves the precision of evaluating operative indications, while facilitating access through concealed incisions. However, by 2 to 3 weeks postinjury, fractures begin to heal, particularly in younger athletes, making accurate reduction more challenging. Most surgeons prefer to operate at 1 to 2 weeks postinjury.[23]

Closed Reduction

Closed reduction has limited indications because of the difficulty of accessing the deep aspect of the midface in the absence of incisions. For isolated zygomatic arch fractures, a bone hook is placed percutaneously over the arch, and a laterally directed force applied to achieve reduction. Similarly, a bone hook, threaded reduction tool (**Fig. 5**A), or screw is applied to the body of the zygoma, and reducing forces applied percutaneously using these tools to reduce ZMC fractures. Many fractures demonstrate inadequate stability or too significant a degree of displacement to be appropriate for these methods. The presence of a fracture along the zygomaticofrontal buttress is predictive of failure of closed reduction, and displacement at this location is an indication for open reduction with internal fixation. Because of the risk of concomitant orbital fracture, forced duction should be completed after closed ZMC reduction to assess for entrapment caused by fracture reduction.

Open Reduction

The number and location of incisions depends on the anticipated sites of fixation. For ZMC fractures, a combination of a lower eyelid and inferior maxillary approach is common, with or without a superolateral approach. For isolated zygomatic arch fractures, the Gilles or Keen approach (described later) provides access for open reduction without fixation. For complex, highly comminuted, or panfacial fractures, or fractures in which osteosynthesis is required along the zygomatic arch, a coronal approach is necessary.

Minimally Invasive Incisions

Isolated zygomatic arch fractures are treated with open reduction via a limited access approach using the Gilles or Keen incisions. The Gilles approach is achieved by making a 2-cm incision within the temporal scalp, 2.5 cm superior and anterior to the helical root (**Fig. 6**A). Use of electric cautery should be minimized to avoid alopecia. Careful palpation prevents incising over the course of the superficial temporal artery. The scalp and subcutaneous tissue are incised. The subcutaneous tissue is bluntly divided until the temporalis fascia is seen (see **Fig. 6**B). The temporalis fascia is incised, exposing the temporalis muscle (see **Fig. 6**C). At this point, an elevator is placed deep to the temporalis fascia, and a sweeping motion allows the elevator to pass caudally, until the tip is deep to the zygomatic arch (see **Fig. 6**D). Applying a laterally directed force while palpating along the arch, the depressed segment is reduced.

In the Keen incision, a 2-cm incision is made in the upper buccal sulcus in the region of the zygomaticomaxillary buttress (**Fig. 7**A–B). An elevator is directed just medial to the arch (see **Fig. 7**C). Laterally directed force with manual palpation guides the completion of reduction.

The stability of the reduced zygomatic arch depends on the fracture location, pattern, and

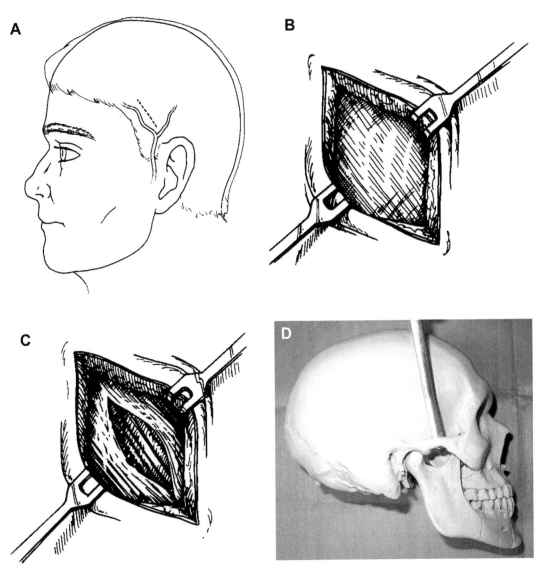

Fig. 6. (*A-D*) The Gilles approach. (*From* Haug RH, Buchbinder D. Incisions for access to craniomaxillofacial fractures. *Atlas Oral Maxillofac Surg Clin North Am*. 1993;1:1–29; with permission)

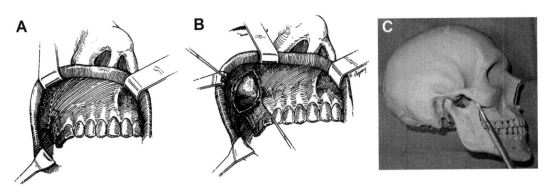

Fig. 7. (*A-C*) The Keen approach. (*From* Haug RH, Buchbinder D. Incisions for access to craniomaxillofacial fractures. *Atlas Oral Maxillofac Surg Clin North Am*. 1993;1:1–29; with permission)

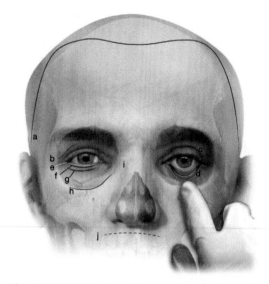

Fig. 8. Selected incisions for periorbital and midface skeletal access include the coronal (a), Wright (b), upper lid crease (c), transconjunctival (d), lateral canthotomy (e), subcilliary (f), subtarsal/mid-lid (g), infraorbital (h), Lynch (i), and upper buccal sulcus (j). (*From* Jones CM, van Aalst JA. Facial fractures and soft tissue injuries. In: Chung K, ed. *Grabb & Smith's Plastic Surgery.* 8th Ed. Wolters Kluwer;2020:1237–1285; with permission)

degree of comminution. Only fractures with a high level of stability should be selected. More comminuted and unstable zygomatic arch fractures, particularly those causing significant aesthetic deformities, may be better suited to open reduction with internal fixation via coronal approach, or later camouflage with bone graft, fat graft, or alloplastic material.

Open Reduction with Internal Fixation

Depending on fracture comminution and concomitant injuries, anterior or posterior approaches may be selected (**Fig. 8**). Anterior approaches allow regional access, and multiple incisions are typically performed depending on the ease of assessing reduction and the number of sites planned for osteosynthesis. The anterior approaches include the lateral brow incisions, upper blepharoplasty or lower eyelid incisions, and upper buccal sulcus incisions. The primary posterior approach is the coronal incision.

The lateral brow incision is a small incision made inferior to the lateral portion of the eyebrow (**Fig. 9**), providing local access to the zygomaticofrontal suture. The incision is made outside the hair-bearing skin to avoid alopecia. The upper blepharoplasty incision is drawn in a supratarsal crease along the lateral portion of the upper eyelid. A skin-muscle flap is elevated, leaving the orbital septum intact, and blunt dissection proceeds in a supraperiosteal plane until the lateral orbital rim is reached. This incision provides access to the lateral orbital wall and zygomaticofrontal suture. The upper blepharoplasty incision is generally preferred over the lateral brow incision.

Lower eyelid incisions include transconjunctival preseptal, transconjunctival postseptal, subcilliary, or infraorbital approaches (**Fig. 10**). These approaches are discussed in detail by Flynn and colleagues in this issue. At the infraorbital rim, subperiosteal dissection proceeds caudally onto the zygoma and medially and laterally along the inferior and lateral orbital rims to expose fracture lines.

The upper buccal sulcus incision is made from the lateral incisor to the first molar, 3 to 4 mm above the mucogingival line to facilitate closure. The position of the parotid duct orifice is checked

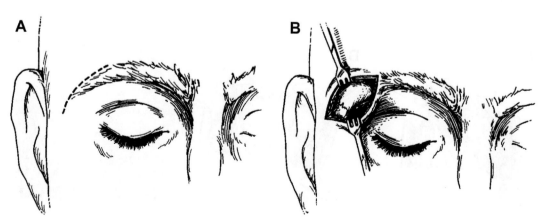

Fig. 9. (*A-B*) The lateral brow incision. (*From* Haug RH, Buchbinder D. Incisions for access to craniomaxillofacial fractures. *Atlas Oral Maxillofac Surg Clin North Am.* 1993;1:1–29; with permission)

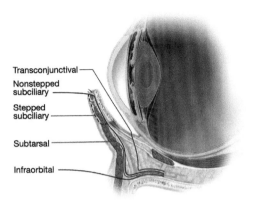

Fig. 10. Cross-sectional view of lower eyelid approaches. (*From* Jones CM, van Aalst JA. Facial fractures and soft tissue injuries. In: Chung K, ed. *Grabb & Smith's Plastic Surgery*. 8th Ed. Wolters Kluwer;2020:1237–1285; with permission)

to avoid injury. After incising the mucosa sharply or with electrocautery, dissection is carried directly down to and through the periosteum. Dissection then switches to a blunt subperiosteal elevation

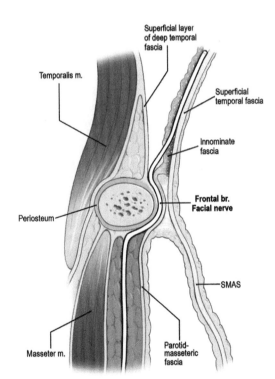

Fig. 11. Anatomy of the temporal region as related to approaches to the zygomatic arch. SMAS, superficial musculoaponeurotic system. (*From* Agarwal CA, Mendenhall SD, Foreman KB, Owsley JQ. The course of the frontal branch of the facial nerve in relation to fascial planes: An anatomic study. *Plast Reconstr Surg*. 2010;125:532–537; with permission)

along the nasomaxillary and posterior maxillary buttresses, just medial and lateral to the infraorbital nerve, respectively.

The coronal approach has the advantage of wide exposure of the frontal bone, orbit, malar eminence, and zygomatic arch, and is used to treat a variety of complex facial fractures. However, potential disadvantages include a long scar, alopecia, temporal hollowing, or injury to the frontal branch of the facial nerve. The scar is made less conspicuous by a curving zig-zag pattern, which allows the hair follicles to lie at an angle to the scar. The incision is extended anterior to the helical root in the preauricular crease. A hemicoronal incision is used to access a unilateral zygomaticomaxillary fracture.

The coronal incision is made sharply through the skin, subcutaneous tissue, and galea aponeurotica. Working in small sections, needle-point electrocautery is used to cauterize small vessels while protecting the hair follicles. Avoiding compressive hemostatic clips can minimize alopecia. A subgaleal or supraperiosteal dissection is completed to the supraorbital rims and the superior temporal line. At the superior temporal line, dissection proceeds toward the zygomatic arch along the superficial aspect of the temporalis fascia. Caudally, the yellow outline of the superficial temporal fat pad is seen; at this point, the temporalis fascia splits into the superficial and deep layers of the deep temporal fascia. The superficial layer of the deep temporal fascia is incised, and dissection continues along the deep aspect of this layer, just superficial to the temporal fat pad, using minimal electrocautery to preserve the temporal fat pad. Once the arch is reached, the periosteum is incised, providing access for exposure in the subperiosteal plane. This manner of dissection protects the frontal branch of the facial nerve, which runs superficial to the deep temporal fascia over the zygomatic arch (**Fig. 11**).

Osteosynthesis

Points of fixation

One-, two-, three-, or four-point fixation is selected depending on fracture displacement and comminution.[1,24,28] Titanium plates demonstrate a low complication profile and excellent biomechanical stability and are favored over bioabsorbable plates in most fractures.[2,29,30]

For stable fractures with mild displacement, including minimal to no displacement at the zygomaticofrontal suture, single-point fixation is performed at the posterior maxillary buttress via upper buccal sulcus approach. After elevation of the fracture, an L-shaped plate is placed along

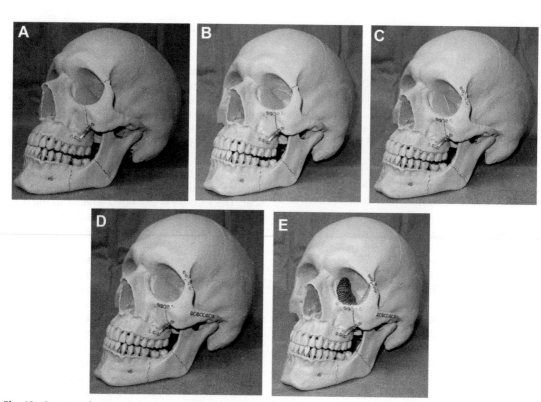

Fig. 12. Osteosynthesis with (*A*) 1-point fixation, (*B*) 2-point fixation, (*C*) 3-point fixation, (*D*) 4-point fixation, and (*E*) 4-point fixation with repair of orbital floor.

the zygomaticomaxillary buttress (**Fig. 12**A). The plate is adapted to the three-dimensional skeletal contour by curving the cephalad portion out-of-plane and opening in-plane to a more obtuse angle. The vertical and horizontal limbs of the plate are secured to thick, stable bone of the posterior maxillary buttress and the alveolar bone superior to the tooth roots. Inadequate plate adaptation places screws into the thin bone of the maxillary sinus. Fracture comminution along the posterior maxillary buttress is common, and is overcome by selecting an L-plate of a longer length. Plate profiles vary. The posterior maxillary buttress contains thick bone that adds significant stability and has the thick overlying buccal fat pad. For this reason, a thicker plate is advocated in this region.[22,24]

A second or third point of fixation is added along the infraorbital rim and/or zygomaticofrontal suture for fractures demonstrating more displacement and less stability (see **Fig. 12**B–C). Plate location is selected by palpating for bony step-offs, evaluating displacement on imaging, and surgeon preference. The skin and soft tissue in both locations is thin, which can make displaced fracture edges or an implanted plate more easily perceptible. In addition to allowing another site of osteosynthesis, a second access can provide better assessment of three-dimensional fracture reduction. The infraorbital rim is accessed through a lower eyelid incision. The zygomaticofrontal buttress is accessed through a lateral blepharoplasty, lateral brow, or coronal approach. In both locations, a low-profile, curvilinear miniplate is typically selected for fixation. Adequacy of reduction should be sequentially checked at each buttress. A plate is adapted at one fracture first, typically the zygomaticofrontal buttress, using a single screw on either side of the fracture, until adequate reduction and stabilization are achieved at the other visualized sites.

Reduction of the zygomatic bone to the greater wing of the sphenoid should be checked in all but single-point approaches, because it provides the most sensitive evaluation of the adequacy of three-dimensional reduction of the ZMC with the skull base.[24] This is accomplished through the lower eyelid or upper blepharoplasty incision via subperiosteal dissection along the lateral orbital wall. Comminution along the lateral orbital wall makes assessment of the zygomaticosphenoid reduction more difficult, and more emphasis is then placed on evaluating other articulations. Completing osteosynthesis at the zygomaticosphenoid buttress is uncommon because of difficulty obtaining an appropriate angle for fixation.

A fourth point of fixation is added along the zygomatic arch in the most complex, comminuted, or unstable fractures, particularly those causing deformity along the arch (see **Fig. 12**D–E).[2] A coronal approach is needed to access the arch directly. A long miniplate can stabilize multiple fracture segments. This technique has the advantage of excellent visualization of all zygomatic articulations, allowing reduction to be checked sequentially. In general, the zygomaticofrontal buttress provides an initial point of stability, creating a superiorly based hinge, while the other articulations are assessed and stabilized. Beginning with articulations that are least comminuted helps simplify the fracture.

With unstable or highly impacted ZMC fractures, a threaded reduction tool can help reduce the zygoma and add stability while osteosynthesis is completed (see **Fig. 5**A–B).[1] This tool is applied to the body of the zygoma through the lower eyelid incision or directly via percutaneous approach (**Fig. 13**A–D).

Traditionally, the orbital floor was routinely explored after reduction of the ZMC to ensure that it did not need repair. More recently, it has become apparent that this is usually unnecessary and the need to repair is accurately predicted based on the preoperative CT imaging. Alternatively, intraoperative imaging after ZMC reduction can determine whether orbital floor exploration is indicated.[25]

In pediatric athletes who have not yet completed growth, consideration should be given to using absorbable plates and screws when internal fixation is necessary.[5,8,24] Titanium plates can migrate with growth and require secondary removal. In young athletes, fracture at the zygomaticomaxillary buttress is most common, with incomplete greenstick fracture at the zygomaticofrontal buttress. These cases may be treated with intraoral reduction and a single plate placed along the zygomaticomaxillary buttress.[8]

Intraoperative Imaging

Long used in neurosurgical and orthopedic applications, intraoperative CT is becoming more commonly applied to treatment of facial fractures. Properly executed, the scan adds little time to the operation and has been shown to reduce the rate of reoperation by prompting necessary revisions intraoperatively.[31,32] Intraoperative imaging can assess whether an additional approach is needed after single- or two-point fixation of the ZMC.[33]

The use of intraoperative imaging has the ability to change treatment algorithms of concomitant orbital floor fractures. Exploring the orbital floor reduces its stability by releasing periosteal attachments of small bone fragments, increasing the likelihood that fractures need to be treated. Through imaging before exploration, a more accurate assessment of the fracture pattern and size is achieved to tailor treatment to the individual defect.[33,34]

Intraoperative Navigation

Technology widely used in neurosurgery and endoscopic sinus surgery is now being adapted for treatment of craniomaxillofacial trauma.[28] Intraoperative navigation combines preoperative facial scans with intraoperative positioning devices to allow more accurate assessment of reduction. If VSP is conducted preoperatively, the simulated reduction can be uploaded to the navigation system for real-time assessment of plan execution.

Inserting positioning screws onto the maxilla before preoperative CT acquisition provides stable intraoperative reference points (**Fig. 14**A). Preoperative virtual reduction is done via VSP, and the unreduced and reduced scans uploaded to the system (see **Fig. 14**B). Intraoperatively, the patient is fitted with a digital reference frame fixed to the skull with a titanium screw (see **Fig. 14**C). Reference points are marked using an instrument with light-reflecting balls, which reflect infrared rays emitted by cameras (see **Fig. 14**D). By registering the positioning screws, navigation accuracy is checked to less than 1 mm (see **Fig. 14**E).[27,28] Combining VSP, intraoperative navigation, and intraoperative imaging provides an accurate process of planning, execution, and verification of the desired operative result.[1]

POSTOPERATIVE CARE
Routine Care

Patients should elevate the head to reduce edema and pain. If orbital exploration was undertaken, visual acuity should be examined postoperatively. A temporary suture tarsorrhaphy (Frost suture) is commonly used with lower eyelid approaches to manage early chemosis. In this technique, a monofilament suture, such as 4–0 Prolene, is passed through the gray line of the lower tarsal plate and taped to the forehead. The suture is removed once the risk of severe chemosis has subsided, commonly on the first postoperative day, before discharge. Dry eye is managed with artificial tears during the day and lubricating ointment at night. Nose-blowing is avoided for about 10 days to avoid orbital emphysema and propagation of sinus bacteria into the orbital soft tissue.[35] Oral hygiene with regular brushing of teeth and

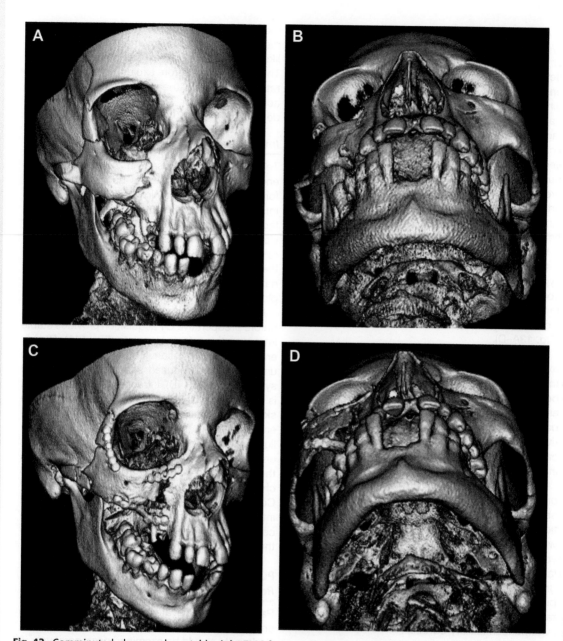

Fig. 13. Comminuted, depressed, unstable right ZMC fracture (*A, B*) was treated with 3-point fixation (*C, D*). This is the same patient demonstrated in **Figs. 4 and 5**B.

use of chlorhexidine mouthwash is prescribed for at least 2 weeks. Following a soft diet for the first 2 to 4 weeks reduces pain related to exertion of the muscles of mastication.

Complications

Inadequate reduction of zygomaticomaxillary fractures can lead to continued deformity or trismus.[36] This is prevented through the use of intraoperative imaging or detected early with postoperative CT before discharge. Significant residual displacement

may require reoperation. Late-presenting patients with history of ZMC malunion may benefit from osteotomies or skeletal camouflage with bone graft, alloplastic malar implants, and/or fat grafting. The widening of the midface characteristic of ZMC fracture is more difficult to camouflage and may require osteotomies for proper reduction.

Infraorbital hypoesthesia is accentuated by traction injury during the operative approach. Dysesthesia is persistent in up to 50% of patients.[33,36]

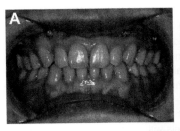
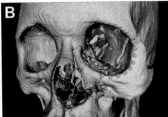
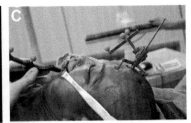
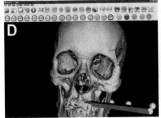
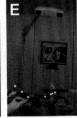

Fig. 14. (*A-E*) Intraoperative navigation. (*From* Yu H, Shen G, Wang Z, Zhang S. Navigation-guided reduction and orbital floor reconstruction in the treatment of zygomatic-orbital-maxillary complex fractures. J Oral Maxillofac Surg. 2010;68:28–34; with permission)

Intraoral incisional dehiscence can lead to hardware exposure at the zygomaticomaxillary buttress. The oral cavity often remucosalizes; re-exploration and closure may be undertaken if dehiscence occurs in the early postoperative period. Ectropion can occur from lower eyelid approaches, with the subcilliary approach demonstrating the highest incidence. Mild ectropion often resolves with massage; more severe cases may require operative intervention.

Redraping of the soft tissues is critical to prevent midfacial descent. In the lower eyelid approach, the midfacial periosteum is resuspended to the infraorbital rim or hardware.[37] Failure to adequately resuspend the soft tissue can lead to ectropion, premature aging, corneal exposure, and epiphora.[24] In the coronal approach, the temporoparietal fascia is reapproximated to prevent temporal hollowing.[1]

Failure to recognize or adequately treat a concomitant orbital floor fracture can lead to enophthalmos, reduction in the palpebral fissure with pseudoptosis, and diplopia.[2] Operative treatment of the orbital fracture is required to resolve these complaints.

The hardware placed along the alveolar ridge at the zygomaticomaxillary buttress should be positioned just cephalad to the tooth roots. Inadvertent injury to tooth roots can occur, requiring specialized dental treatment to avoid chronic infection and loss of the tooth. The hardware at the infraorbital rim or zygomaticofrontal can become palpable but is rarely visible. Hardware at any site uncommonly requires removal for these or other indications.

CLINICS CARE POINTS

- Displacement of the ZMC or zygomatic arch can cause functional and aesthetic concerns, and is the primary indication for operative management.

- The choice of the number of access incisions and points of fixation seeks to balance morbidity of the exposures with stability of osteosynthesis. Only the exposures that are necessary for a given fracture are performed.

- Excessive traction on the infraorbital nerve should be avoided to reduce long-term hypoesthesia.

DISCLOSURE STATEMENT

C. Schmalbach: Teaching honorarium for AO North America CMF, nonprofit teaching consortium.

C. Jones: None.

REFERENCES

1. Strong EB, Gary C. Management of zygomaticomaxillary complex fractures. Facial Plast Surg Clin North Am 2017;25:547–62.
2. Kelley P, Crawford M, Higuera S, et al. Two hundred ninety-four consecutive facial fractures in an urban trauma center: lessons learned. Plast Reconstr Surg 2005;116:42e–9e.

3. MacIsaac ZM, Berhane H, Cray J, et al. Nonfatal sport-related craniofacial fractures: characteristics, mechanisms, and demographic data in the pediatric population. Plast Reconstr Surg 2013;131:1339–47.

4. Salehi PP, Heiser A, Torabi SJ, et al. Facial fractures and the National Basketball Association: epidemiology and outcomes. Laryngoscope 2020;130:E824–32.

5. Fujisawa K, Suzuki A, Yamakawa T, et al. Pediatric-specific midfacial fracture patterns and management: pediatric versus adult patients. J Craniofac Surg 2020;31:e312–5.

6. Naran S, MacIsaac Z, Katzel E, et al. Pediatric craniofacial fractures: trajectories and ramifications. J Craniofac Surg 2016;27:1535–8.

7. Ghosh R, Gopalkrishnan K, Anand J. Pediatric facial fractures: a 10-year study. J Maxillofac Oral Surg 2018;17:158–63.

8. Eppley BL. Use of resorbable plates and screws in pediatric facial fractures. J Oral Maxillofac Surg 2005;63:385–91.

9. Dobitsch AA, Oleck NC, Liu FC, et al. Sports-related pediatric facial trauma: analysis of facial fracture pattern and concomitant injuries. Surg J 2019;5:e146–9.

10. Viozzi CF. Maxillofacial and mandibular fractures in sports. Clin Sports Med 2017;36:355–68.

11. Manson PN, Clark N, Robertson B, et al. Subunit principles in midface fractures: the importance of sagittal buttresses, soft-tissue reductions, and sequencing treatment of segmental fractures. Plast Reconstr Surg 1999;103:1287–306.

12. Timashpolsky A, Dagum AB, Sayeed SM, et al. A prospective analysis of physical examination findings in the diagnosis of facial fractures: determining predictive value. Plast Surg (Oakv) 2016;24:73–9.

13. Chang CM, Ko EC, Kao CC, et al. Incidence and clinical significance of zygomaticomaxillary complex fracture involving the temporomandibular joint with emphasis on trismus. Kaohsiung J Med Sci 2012;28:336–40.

14. Tahernia A, Erdmann D, Follmar K, et al. Clinical implications of orbital volume change in the management of isolated and zygomaticomaxillary complex-associated orbital floor injuries. Plast Reconstr Surg 2009;123:968–75.

15. Elzanie AS, Park KE, Irgebay Z, et al. Zygoma fractures are associated with increased morbidity and mortality in the pediatric population. J Craniofac Surg 2021;32:559–63.

16. Halsey JN, Hoppe IC, Marano AA, et al. Characteristics of cervical spine injury in pediatric patients with facial fractures. J Craniofac Surg 2016;27:109–11.

17. Maurer P, Conrad-Hengerer I, Hollisten S, et al. Orbital haemorrhage associated with orbital fractures in geriatric patients on antiplatelet or anticoagulant therapy. Int J Oral Maxillofac Surg 2013;42:1510–4.

18. Jamal BT, Diecidue RJ, Taub D, et al. Orbital hemorrhage and compressive optic neuropathy in patients with midfacial fractures receiving low-molecular weight heparin therapy. J Oral Maxillofac Surg 2009;67:1416–9.

19. Jamal BT, Pfahler SM, Lane KA, et al. Ophthalmic injuries in patients with zygomaticomaxillary complex fractures requiring surgical repair. J Oral Maxillofac Surg 2009;67:986–9.

20. Malik AH, Shah AA, Ahmad I, et al. Ocular injuries in patients of zygomatico-complex (ZMC) fractures. J Maxillofac Oral Surg 2017;16:243–7.

21. Hopper RA, Salemy S, Sze RW. Diagnosis of midface fractures with CT: what the surgeon needs to know. Radiographics 2006;26:783–93.

22. Manson PN, Markowitz B, Mirvis S, et al. Toward CT-based facial fracture treatment. Plast Reconstr Surg 1990;85:202–12.

23. Birgfeld CB, Mundinger GS, Gruss JS. Evidence-based medicine: evaluation and treatment of zygoma fractures. Plast Reconstr Surg 2016;139:168e–80e.

24. Lee EI, Mohan K, Koshy JC, et al. Optimizing the surgical management of zygomaticomaxillary complex fractures. Semin Plast Surg 2010;24:389–97.

25. Flynn J, Lu GN, Kriet JD, et al. Trends in concurrent orbital floor repair during zygomaticomaxillary complex fracture repair. JAMA Facial Plast Surg 2019;21(4):341–3.

26. Tel A, Sembronio S, Costa F, et al. Scoping zygomaticomaxillary complex fractures with the eyes of virtual reality: operative protocol and proposal of a modernized classification. J Craniofac Surg 2021;32:552–8.

27. Yu H, Shen G, Wang Z, et al. Navigation-guided reduction and orbital floor reconstruction in the treatment of zygomatic-orbital-maxillary complex fractures. J Oral Maxillofac Surg 2010;68:28–34.

28. Zhang Z, Ye L, Li H, et al. Surgical navigation improves reductions accuracy of unilateral complicated zygomaticomaxillary complex fractures: a randomized controlled trial. Sci Rep 2018;8:6890.

29. Jazayeri HE, Khavanin N, Yu JW, et al. Fixation points in the treatment of traumatic zygomaticomaxillary complex fractures: a systematic review and meta-analysis. J Oral Maxillofac Surg 2019;77:2064–73.

30. Kasrai L, Hearn T, Gur E, et al. A biomechanical analysis of the orbitozygomatic complex in human cadavers: examination of load sharing and failure patterns following fixation with titanium and bioresorbable plating systems. J Craniofac Surg 1999;10:237–43.

31. Shaye DA, Tollefson TT, Strong EB. Use of intraoperative computed tomography for maxillofacial

reconstructive surgery. JAMA Facial Plast Surg 2015;17:113–9.

32. Alasraj A, Alasseri N, Al-Moraissi E. Does intraoperative computed tomography scanning in maxillofacial trauma surgery affect the revision rate? J Oral Maxillofac Surg 2021;79:214–419.

33. Wilde F, Lorenz K, Ebner AK, et al. Intraoperative imaging with a 3D C-arm system after zygomatic-orbital complex fracture reduction. J Oral Maxillofac Surg 2013;71:894–910.

34. Borad V, Lacey MS, Hamlar DD, et al. Intraoperative imaging changes management in orbital fracture repair. J Oral Maxillofac Surg 2017;75:1932–40.

35. Cornelius CP, Gellrich N, Hillerup S, et al. Zygoma, zygomatic complex fracture. AO Surgery Reference website. Available at: https://surgeryreference. aofoundation.org/cmf/trauma/midface/zygomatic-complex-fracture. [Accessed 29 March 2021].

36. Kurita M, Okazaki M, Ozaki M, et al. Patient satisfaction after open reduction and internal fixation of zygomatic bone fractures. J Craniofac Surg 2010; 21:45–9.

37. Phillips JH, Gruss JS, Wells MD, et al. Periosteal suspension of the lower eyelid and cheek following subciliary exposure of facial fractures. Plast Reconstr Surg 1991;88:145–8.

Midface Including Le Fort Level Injuries

Katherine A. Larrabee, MD[a],*, Andrew S. Kao, MS[b], Benjamin T. Barbetta, DMD, MD[c], Lamont R. Jones, MD, MBA[a],*

KEYWORDS

- Facial trauma • Athletic injuries • Le fort fractures • Midface injuries

KEY POINTS

- Le Fort fractures occur at uniform weak areas in the midface often due to a blunt impact to the face.
- Sporting injuries are a common cause of facial trauma; however, use of protective equipment has reduced the number of sports-related craniofacial injuries.
- Le Fort fractures can contribute to airway obstruction and urgent intubation may be indicated.
- Surgery is indicated for most displaced Le Fort fractures to restore function and facial harmony. Good exposure is critical. The patient is placed in maxillomandibular fixation (MMF) to facilitate reduction and establish the original occlusive relationship. The sequence of fracture repair is variable.

INTRODUCTION

Le Fort level fractures are complex facial fractures that are differentiated as I, II, and III based on fracture patterns. The location of the injury, velocity and energy transfer at impact, and patient-related factors determine the fracture severity and pattern. Le Fort fractures typically occur due to blunt impact to the midface. Motor vehicle accidents (MVAs), interpersonal violence, industrial accidents, falls, and sports-related injuries are common mechanisms of injury. Sporting injuries account for 10% to 42% of all facial fractures, with midface fractures accounting for a large percentage of these injuries.[1,2] In recent years, there has been a rise in craniofacial injuries related to motor scooters with the introduction of electronic scooters to many cities. Studies noted significant bony injury to the midface with these fractures.[3–5]

Facial fractures due to sporting injuries are generally less severe than those caused by MVAs and are associated with shorter hospitalization time.[6] Le Fort level fractures are more common in high-velocity sports such as mountain biking or skiing.[7] Sporting fracture mechanisms typically include player–player collisions and impact from equipment such as a ball–face impact with improper protective equipment.[8,9] This chapter reviews pertinent anatomy, initial patient workup, and principles of surgical repair with an emphasis on Le Fort pattern fractures related to sports.

Preventing Injuries with Protective Equipment

The use of protective equipment in sports such as helmets, facemasks, and intraoral mouthguards has significantly reduced the number of craniofacial injuries.[8,9] Although traditional helmets have been shown to reduce cranial injuries, they leave the mid and lower face unprotected. Studies are needed to determine if helmets with an extension to cover the lower jaw reduce the prevalence of mid and lower facial injuries. One study found that baseball players using faceguards were 35% less likely to suffer facial injuries than nonusers.[10]

[a] Department of Otolaryngology HNS, DETC K8 Clinic, Henry Ford Hospital 2799 E Grand Boulevard, Detroit, MI 48202, USA; [b] Wayne State University School of Medicine, 540 E Canfield St, Detroit, MI 48201, USA; [c] Division of Oral & Maxillofacial Surgery, DETC K8 Clinic, Henry Ford Hospital 2799 E Grand Boulevard, Detroit, MI 48202, USA
* Corresponding author.
E-mail addresses: klarrab1@hfhs.org (K.A.L.); ljones5@hfhs.org (L.R.J.)

Facial Plast Surg Clin N Am 30 (2022) 63–70
https://doi.org/10.1016/j.fsc.2021.08.005

Mouthguards may act as impact absorption devices which distribute energy from a traumatic blow in order to prevent direct force on oral structures and reduce trauma from mandible and maxilla contact.[9] Recent increases in craniofacial trauma due to motor scooter use have been associated with noncompliance with the safety requirements and to lack of head and facial safety equipment.[4,5]

Anatomic Considerations

The maxilla, a critical part of the human viscerocranium, is formed by the fusion of two pyramid-shaped maxillary bones at the palatine process. This fusion creates the main horizontal buttress of the face. The development of the maxilla provides support to the orbit, houses the maxillary sinus and maxillary dentition, and creates a "crumple zone" as kinetic energy in blunt force trauma is passed through the skeleton protecting the brain and neurocranium posteriorly.

The maxilla consists of the maxillary body and the frontal, zygomatic, palatine and alveolar processes. Energy delivered upon impact to the maxilla will transfer through the bone to the pyriform rim, zygoma, and pterygoid plates. These vertical buttresses absorb and distribute masticatory forces from the teeth to the skull base. There are three paired vertical buttresses: nasomaxillary (medial), zygomaticomaxillary (lateral), and pterygomaxillary (posterior). A fourth, single buttress, the nasal septum, exists at the midline (Fig. 1B). Although the vertical buttresses provide support and structure, they are susceptible to damage from transverse forces. The vertical buttresses are reinforced by three horizontal buttresses: the superior and inferior orbital rims and the alveolar ridge. The pterygoid plates provide posterior support to the maxilla.

This complicated developmental conjugation of the midface creates uniform weak areas prone to fractures in specific patterns (see Fig. 1A). These patterns were initially classified by René Le Fort in 1901 with a classification system that is still used today.[11] Le Fort fractures are described as either unilateral or bilateral.

Le Fort I fracture lines are superficial to the alveolar ridge and create a separation through the maxillary sinus wall horizontally with disjunction of the maxilla from the pterygoid plate (Fig. 2B). Le Fort II fractures are pyramid-shaped central midface fractures that include extension superiomedially through the nasal bones, nasal process of the frontal bone or nasion, medial orbital walls, and inferior orbital rim (see Fig. 2C). Le Fort III fractures result in complete disjunction of the maxilla

from the skull base due to a transverse fracture extending from the pterygoid plate superiorly to the zygomaticofrontal suture, horizontally through the orbit to the nasofrontal suture (see Figs. 2A, B). These are the most severe type of Le Fort fractures and carry additional risk of blindness secondary to the fracture extension near the optic nerve.

Initial Evaluation

All patients who present to the hospital with traumatic injuries should be evaluated using Advanced Trauma Life Support (ATLS) protocol. The primary goals of the ATLS protocol include securing a stable airway, supporting ventilation, evaluating circulation, identifying and controlling life-threatening hemorrhage, obtaining a baseline neurologic evaluation, and exposing the patient to evaluate for injuries. Life-threatening injuries, including intracranial, spinal, and visceral injuries, require urgent attention. Le Fort fractures can contribute to airway obstruction secondary to hemorrhage, posterior inferior displacement of the maxilla, oropharyngeal edema, and hematoma.[12,13] As many as 31% of patients with Le Fort fractures require intubation or tracheotomy due to airway obstruction or acute respiratory failure.[14] Cervical spine instability/injury must also be taken into consideration. Standardized clinical and radiographic protocols should be implemented for workup and management of cervical spine injury. Intubation with a fiberoptic scope may be indicated. In rare instances, blunt cerebrovascular injury (BCVI) can occur with high impact craniomaxillofacial injuries.[15] Computed tomography angiography is the recommended imaging modality to evaluate for these injuries. Plain X-ray films are mostly historical and inadequate to evaluate midfacial fractures.

Once the patient has been stabilized and initial survey is complete a complete history and physical examination should be obtained. History of present illness can be challenging to obtain. It is critical to use all available resources including previous hospital records, first responder accounts of the trauma scene, and family/witnesses. Understanding the mechanism of injury, including the vector and severity of the force, can help predict the involved structures. Mechanism of injury can also provide extremely valuable information about the cleanliness of the wound and potential for foreign bodies. The patient's history can further direct additional workup which can be lifesaving.

Midface edema and ecchymosis are common with midface trauma and can make evaluation

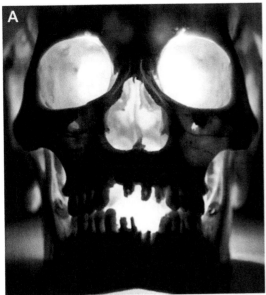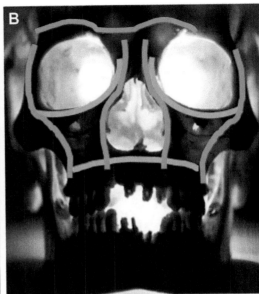

Fig. 1. (*A*) Light shines through the skull illuminating weak points in the midface skeleton that correspond with Le Fort patterns of fractures. (*B*) Vertical (green) and horizontal (blue) buttress system.

for facial symmetry and bony step-offs challenging. Evaluation for midface mobility can be accomplished by stabilizing the cranium while grasping the maxillary alveolar ridge. Intubation can make evaluation of the stability of the maxilla challenging as tube holding devices can stabilize the teeth and fracture. Anterior open bite malocclusion may indicate displacement of the maxillary segment due to caudal pull by the medial pterygoid muscles. The palate should be examined via direct visualization and palpation to identify palatal fractures and lacerations. Palatal fractures can create maxillary width discrepancies that present as a crossbite when the patient is brought into occlusion. Additionally, large palatal lacerations should be identified as typical repair of the Le Fort fractures includes access to the midface via the maxillary vestibule. This access, along with separation of the septum, and possible laceration of the descending palatine arteries creates a situation where the ascending pharyngeal artery is the sole blood supply of the maxilla. Failure to recognize lacerations in this area before surgical access could predispose patients to avascular necrosis. The clinician should inspect for missing or loose teeth and tooth sockets. Any missing teeth with evidence of avulsion should be accounted for. If unable to account for missing teeth, then it is recommended to review computerized tomography (CT) imaging of the face to evaluate for teeth dislodged to other areas. Additionally, an AP chest X-ray is recommended to confirm that there was no aspiration during the injury. A comprehensive ophthalmologic examination should be performed especially in Le Fort II-III type fracture patterns. In addition, evaluation for cerebrospinal fluid leak should also be included when midface fractures occur jointly with skull base injuries.

Diagnostic Imaging

The excellent resolution of CT and the availability of three-dimensional (3D) reconstruction have made CT scanning the method of choice for evaluating complex facial fractures.[16] With current technology, fine-cut CT is a largely preferred modality as this will provide detail necessary to fully visualize the complexity of the trauma and provide enough data to use 3D imaging and 3D printing technology if desired. The ideal resolution is <0.1 mm which can be achieved by modern cone beam computed tomography imaging; hospital CTs should routinely be able to provide <1 mm slices which is acceptable. Vertical and horizontal structures are viewed best on axial and coronal views, respectively.[17] A methodical and thorough evaluation is important in order to accurately diagnose midface fractures. MRI may be used to evaluate soft tissue, intracranial, and vascular injuries, but it has limited usefulness in evaluating skeletal injuries. Imaging of the brain and cervical spine and neck vessels should be performed to evaluate for BCVI with CTA. This is critical for severe injuries or when involvement of vessels is suspected.

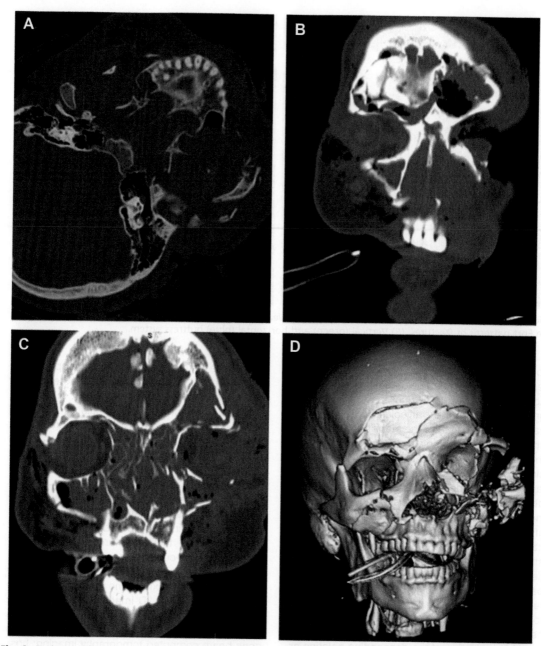

Fig. 2. Patient with extensive facial fractures after motor vehicle accident. (*A*) Axial CT scan in bone window showing Le Fort III injury with fracture through the pterygoid plate as well as the right zygoma. (*B*) Coronal CT scan in bone window showing bilateral Le Fort level I and III fractures. (*C*) Bilateral Le Fort level II fracture as well as orbital floor and palate fractures. (*D*) 3D reconstruction of CT scan showing extensive injuries.

Surgical Indications

Surgery is indicated for a majority of displaced Le Fort fractures, especially those that impact form and/or function. Nondisplaced and minimally displaced fractures that do not affect function and/or cause facial disharmony can be managed conservatively with or without protective devices.

Goals of fracture repair include restoration of occlusion secondary to maligned maxilla or restricted mandibular movement because of coronoid process impingement. Surgical repair can also facilitate a clean, stable, well-approximated midface skeleton which is critical for bony union.[4,18,19] The restoration of preinjury facial harmony is an indication for surgery. In the athlete, an important goal is typically safe and timely return to play; the need for open or closed surgical intervention can impact when an athlete can return to competition.

Indications for closed surgical treatment, such as maxillary mandibular fixation, include nondisplaced, nonmobile fractures in reliable patients who can follow-up for monitoring. Closed surgical treatment often minimizes pain and facilitates return to preinjury occlusion during the healing period. Open surgical treatment, also known as open reduction and internal fixation, is indicated for complex fractures that result in malocclusion, disruption of facial harmony, and are associated with neurologic complication such as visual disturbances and cerebrospinal fluid leakage. In general, open reduction requires longer downtime compared with closed approaches.

Surgical Approach: Airway

When possible, nasotracheal intubation is ideal, as it optimizes exposure and allows for establishment of premorbid occlusion following maxillomandibular fixation (MMF). Retromolar and submental intubations are alternatives to nasotracheal intubation that allow occlusion to be evaluated intraoperatively. In the event of significant skull base injuries, severe facial deformities, anticipated prolonged intubation, or expected multiple returns to the operating room, tracheotomy may be preferred.

Surgical Approach: Exposure

Good exposure is critical for a successful repair. All fractures should be visible before stabilization.[19] Access can sometimes be accomplished through existing facial lacerations. The entire anterior maxilla including the zygomaticomaxillary buttress, the infraorbital foramen and nerve, orbital rim, and piriform aperture can be accessed through a maxillary vestibular incision. This incision alone is often adequate for Le Fort level I injuries. A coronal incision may be required in more extensive fracture cases and readily provides exposure of the nasal root and supraorbital rims. The incision can be extended to access the zygomatic arch and bilateral zygomas if necessary. Limited access to the zygomaticofrontal suture can be obtained with a lateral brow or upper blepharoplasty incision. The orbital floor and infraorbital rim can also be accessed via a transconjunctival, subciliary, or infraorbital skin incision.

Surgical Approach: Sequence of Approach and Repair

Once exposure is optimized, the fracture site should be cleaned extensively. Removal of blood products, tissue, and foreign material not only will allow for better adaptation of the bony segments but also will improve the environment for bone healing. Following exposure and cleaning, the bone is ready for reduction under direct visualization. To facilitate reduction in Le Fort fractures, the original occlusive relationship should be restored by placing the patient in MMF. MMF can be established with interdental wiring, intermaxillary fixation screws, conventional arch bars, hybrid arch bars, ivy loops, or using bonded orthodontic hardware.

In these cases, it is imperative that the operative surgeon mobilizes the maxilla to allow for passive seating of the patient into a stable and repeatable occlusal relationship. Using existing wear facets or comparing current occlusion to preoperative photographs can help. It is important to work with the anesthesiologist during this stage of the surgery. The midface is highly vascular, and control of bleeding is often not possible until osteotomies are performed and segments are replaced.[20] Movement of the maxilla, including down fracture, is associated with the highest incidence of bleeding in these cases. In a study of Le Fort I patients, the mean estimated intraoperative blood loss was 945 mL, with 50% of cases reporting greater than 1000 mL.[20] Permissive hypotension can reduce some of the blood loss but should be used with caution in older and medically complex patients.[20] Additionally, muscle paralysis is critical when establishing occlusion as muscle pull can inadvertently create occlusal discrepancies. In cases with unusual premorbid occlusal patterns, segmental fractures of the maxilla, or difficulty establishing intraoperative occlusion, fabrication of an occlusal splint is recommended.

In edentulous patients, if establishment of MMF is desired, it is necessary to use a gunning splint. This can be specifically made for the patient. Alternatively, existing dentures can be modified to accept screws or wire fixation to the jaw and can help establish an appropriate vertical dimension to guide operative efforts if open repair is essential. In addition, osteotomies may be necessary to mobilize the midface when fractures are incomplete or unusual. Palatal fractures generally reduce well once establishing proper occlusion. Palatal fractures can easily be plated on the anterior surface of the maxilla superior/between the tooth roots. The operative surgeon should strongly consider alternative options to creating additional cuts on the palatal mucosa or implanting hardware on the palatal bone. Once the fracture is reduced and the occlusion reestablished, the surgeon can select a fixation technique that allows for stabilization of the bones and realignment of the segments.

For uncomplicated fractures, L-shaped plates at the zygomaticomaxillary buttress and piriform rim should allow for adequate fixation and will be positioned in the best bone stock available to hold the hardware.

The sequence of the approach is surgeon specific, and multiple approaches have been described. The senior author prefers working from the periphery to the center to transform a Le Fort III fracture into a Le Fort II and subsequently into a Le Fort I fracture. This approach of reducing Le Fort fractures from complex to simple allows for an orderly repair of the midface and reestablishes both midface height and width. First, frontal fractures are repaired creating a solid frontal bar. Next, the bizygomatic width must be reconstructed. When the frontal bone is intact and the zygomatic arches are continuous, the midfacial height and bitemporal width are reestablished by repairing the zygomaticofrontal suture. By stabilizing the zygoma to the frontal and temporal bones, a Le Fort III fracture has been reduced to a Le Fort II fracture. Next, the nasofrontal area is repaired, thereby reducing the Le Fort II component and converting it to a Le Fort I fracture.

Virtual Planning and Intraoperative Imaging

There are many challenges when it comes to repairing Le Fort level facial trauma. First, there is the complexity of facial anatomy and importance of restoring function and structure to the facial skeleton with the primary goals being to restore occlusion and obtain bony union which will facilitate proper mastication and speech and minimize pain. Visualizing 3D relationships from a two-dimensional image is a challenge, especially in regions with complex 3D anatomy. It can be difficult to directly view the deep facial skeleton from esthetic incision lines, and it can therefore be difficult to visually assess the intraoperative result for ideal projection and position. Additionally, edema limits evaluation of symmetry. Use of preoperative and intraoperative imaging can help address some of these challenges. With the availability of intraoral scanners, 3D images of the teeth can be obtained and fused with CT imaging. This surface-generated image is not distorted by dental materials like images obtained using ionizing radiation. This allows for more accurate representation of the dentition and occlusion and permits accurate fabrication of planned surgical splints that can recreate a planned occlusion intraoperatively. Image-guided simulation with use of 3D CT allows for preoperative analysis and manipulation of images as part of a comprehensive surgical planning session. Surgeons can then manipulate the fractured segments while observing the effect on reference anatomic structures, compare the fractures to "standard anatomy" or unaffected sides, and create micromovements which are easily reproducible in vivo. Although 3D reconstruction of scans can provide an important tool for the operative surgeon, it is critical that the images be evaluated carefully in the nonreformatted views. Volume averaging in the 3D reconstruction can underestimate fractures and may mislead a surgical team. Nevertheless, surgeons report a subjective preference for viewing images in 3D, and one study shows improved diagnostic accuracy with 3D CT scans.[21]

Another useful tool is intraoperative imaging which allows the surgeon to evaluate the repair in the operating room and make adjustments in real time. This is most useful when positioning fracture segments, grafts, or hardware near vital structures like the optic nerve. Postoperative CT is considered the gold standard for the evaluation of surgical outcomes, but errors identified with this approach would require return to the operating room. New technology allows for more mobile CT scans with rapid processing time and low radiation exposure making intraoperative imaging more realistic.[22] Although the majority of Le Fort fractures are easily visualized with standard surgical approaches and using the as low as reasonably achievable standard for diagnostic imaging and radiation, intraoperative CT can be an extremely useful intraoperative tool when used correctly in limited situations. This technology is increasingly available in operating rooms. The mean total operating time is minimal, and the use of intraoperative CT often results in intraoperative revisions.[22] It is not clear how this relates to patient outcomes, but ultimately, addressing malposition or insufficient reductions intraoperatively results in decreased complication and reoperation rates.[23]

Return to Play

Evidence-based research to establish return-to-play guidelines is limited. Recovery periods of up to 6 weeks have been reported in literature with some advocating return to activity at 3 weeks with graduated participation until 6 weeks.[6,24] Professional athletes are under significant pressure to return to play in a timely manner, but this must be weighted carefully in terms of possibility of reinjury and need for healing from the initial event. Loss of play time can negatively impact position in team and loss of salary. Early return with insufficient time for recover is associated with high risk of another impact to the injured site.[25] The use of sports-orthosis or protective equipment can provide psychological reassurance and may prevent reinjury, but research on the efficacy of these devices is lacking.[25] These advantages must be weighed against their shortcomings, such as obstructing sight, being hot, and uncomfortable, and, in some sports, the appearance of these devices has been not accepted by athletes. The appropriate time to return to play is likely athlete, injury, and sport specific. Sports more prone to repeat injury such as boxing would likely require longer convalescence than sporting with lower contact risk.

CLINICS CARE POINTS

- Le Fort fractures typically occur due to blunt impact to the midface
- Sporting injuries accounts for 10% to 42% of all facial fractures[1]
- Le Fort level fractures are more common in high-velocity sports
- Use of protective equipment reduces the number of craniofacial injuries[8,9]
- The midface has uniform weak areas which are prone to fracturing in specific patterns
- Le Fort I fracture lines result in disjunction of the maxilla from the pterygoid plate
- Le Fort II fractures are pyramid-shaped central midface fractures
- Le Fort III fractures result in complete disjunction of the maxilla from the skull base
- All patients with traumatic injuries should be evaluated using the Advanced Trauma Life Support protocol
- Le Fort fractures can contribute to airway obstruction, and urgent intubation may be indicated
- Computerized tomography (CT) scanning, with resolution less than 1 mm, is the method of choice for evaluating complex facial fractures
- For surgical repair, nasotracheal intubation is ideal, as it optimizes exposure and allows for establishment of premorbid occlusion
- Surgery is indicated for most displaced Le Fort fractures
- Goals of fracture repair include restoration of occlusion, facial harmony, and to facilitate a clean, stable, well-approximated midface skeleton to allow for healing

- Good exposure is critical for a successful repair
- To facilitate reduction in Le Fort fractures, the original occlusive relationship should be restored by placing the patient in maxillomandibular fixation
- Close collaboration with the anesthesiology team is critical for establishing a safe airway, limiting blood loss and ensuring complete muscle relaxation
- The sequence of repair of facial fractures is surgeon specific, and multiple successful approaches have been described
- Intraoral scanners, three-dimensional CT, and image-guided simulation are useful as part of a comprehensive surgical planning session
- For complex fractures, intraoperative CT can be useful in evaluating and addressing malposition or insufficient reductions intraoperatively

DISCLOSURE

The authors have nothing to disclose.

REFERENCES

1. Yamamoto K, Matsusue Y, Horita S, et al. Trends and characteristics of maxillofacial fractures sustained during sports activities in Japan. Dental Traumatol 2018;34(3):151–7.
2. Viozzi CF. Maxillofacial and mandibular fractures in sports. Clin Sports Med 2017;36(2):355–68.
3. Faraji F, Lee JH, Faraji F, et al. Electric scooter craniofacial trauma. Laryngoscope Investig Otolaryngol 2020;5(3):390–5.
4. Kim M, Lee S, Ko DR, et al. Craniofacial and dental injuries associated with stand-up electric scooters. Dent Traumatol 2021;37(2):229–33.
5. Trivedi B, Kesterke MJ, Bhattacharjee R, et al. Craniofacial injuries seen with the introduction of bicycle-share electric scooters in an urban setting. J Oral Maxillofac Surg 2019;77(11):2292–7.
6. Roccia F, Diaspro A, Nasi A, et al. Management of sport-related maxillofacial injuries. J Craniofac Surg 2008;19(2):377–82.
7. Maladière E, Bado F, Meningaud JP, et al. Aetiology and incidence of facial fractures sustained during sports: a prospective study of 140 patients. Int J Oral Maxillofac Surg 2001;30(4):291–5.
8. Ranalli DN. Prevention of craniofacial injuries in football. Dent Clin North Am 1991;35(4):627–45.
9. Tuna EB, Ozel E. Factors affecting sports-related orofacial injuries and the importance of mouthguards. Sports Med 2014;44(6):777–83.

10. Exadaktylos AK, Eggensperger NM, Eggli S, et al. Sports related maxillofacial injuries: the first maxillofacial trauma database in Switzerland. Br J Sports Med 2004;38(6):750–3.

11. Tessier P. The classic reprint. Experimental study of fractures of the upper jaw. I and II. René Le Fort, M.D. Plast Reconstr Surg 1972;50(5):497–506.

12. Kellman RM, Losquadro WD. Comprehensive airway management of patients with maxillofacial trauma. Craniomaxillofac Trauma Reconstr 2008;1(1):39–47.

13. Ng M, Saadat D, Sinha UK. Managing the emergency airway in Le Fort fractures. J Craniomaxillofac Trauma 1998;4(4):38–43.

14. Thompson JN, Gibson B, Kohut RI. Airway obstruction in LeFort fractures. Laryngoscope 1987;97(3 Pt 1):275–9.

15. Kelts G, Maturo S, Couch ME, et al. Blunt cerebrovascular injury following craniomaxillofacial fractures: a systematic review. Laryngoscope 2017;127(1):79–86.

16. Chen WJ, Yang YJ, Fang YM, et al. Identification and classification in le fort type fractures by using 2D and 3D computed tomography. Chin J Traumatol 2006;9(1):59–64.

17. Levy RA, Rosenbaum AE, Kellman RM, et al. Assessing whether the plane of section on CT affects accuracy in demonstrating facial fractures in 3-D reconstruction when using a dried skull. AJNR Am J Neuroradiol 1991;12(5):861–6.

18. Handler SD. Diagnosis and management of maxillofacial injuries. In: Torg JS, editor. Athletic injuries to the head, neck and face. Philadelphia, PA: Lea & Febiger; 1982. p. 231–44.

19. Phillips BJ, Turco LM. Le fort fractures: a collective review. Bull Emerg Trauma 2017;5(4):221–30.

20. Schaberg SJ, Kelly JF, Terry BC, et al. Blood loss and hypotensive anesthesia in oral-facial corrective surgery. J Oral Surg 1976;34(2):147–56.

21. Reuben AD, Watt-Smith SR, Dobson D, et al. A comparative study of evaluation of radiographs, CT and 3D reformatted CT in facial trauma: what is the role of 3D? Br J Radiol 2005;78(927):198–201.

22. Shaye DA, Tollefson TT, Strong EB. Use of intraoperative computed tomography for maxillofacial reconstructive surgery [published correction appears in JAMA Facial Plast Surg. 2015 May-Jun;17(3):227]. JAMA Facial Plast Surg 2015;17(2):113–9.

23. Andrades P, Maripangui M, Jara R, et al. Intraoperative Fluoroscopy Reduces Complication and Reoperation Rate in Facial Fractures [published online ahead of print, 2020 Sep 8]. Facial Plast Surg Aesthet Med 2020. https://doi.org/10.1089/fpsam.2020.0274.

24. Fowell CJ, Earl P. Return-to-play guidelines following facial fractures. Br J Sports Med 2013;47(10):654–6. https://doi.org/10.1136/bjsports-2012-091697.

25. Ghoseiri K, Ghoseiri G, Bavi A, et al. Face-protective orthosis in sport-related injuries. Prosthet Orthot Int 2013;37(4):329–31. https://doi.org/10.1177/0309364612463929.

Frontal Sinus Fractures
A Contemporary Approach in the Endoscopic Era

Steven G. Hoshal, MD[a], Raj D. Dedhia, MD[b], E. Bradley Strong, MD[a],*

KEYWORDS

• Frontal sinus fractures • Endoscopic approach • Skull base • Cranialization • Camouflage

KEY POINTS

• A lack of clinic evidence results in continued controversy over optimal treatment strategies for frontal sinus fractures.
• Despite a paucity of evidence, logical and effective treatment decisions can be made based on the structural integrity of three anatomic parameters: anterior table, frontal sinus outflow tract, and the posterior table/dura.
• The literature supports a paradigm shift from aggressive, open surgical management to a more conservative treatment algorithm emphasizing observation and minimally invasive endoscopic techniques.
• Long-term follow-up for complex frontal sinus injuries is critical.

INTRODUCTION

The frontal sinus is protected by the thick cortical bone, making frontal sinus fractures relatively uncommon. However, the potential for long-term sequelae is significant, and a comprehensive treatment strategy is critical. Management of these injuries remains controversial,[1] but most authors agree that management should include treatment of intracranial injuries, avoidance of long-term complications, reestablishment of the frontal bone contour, and return of sinus function whenever possible. This chapter provides a comprehensive, evidence-based algorithm for management of these injuries in the endoscopic era.

ANATOMY AND EPIDEMIOLOGY

The frontal sinus is absent at birth. A rudimentary cavity develops by 1 to 2 years of age, and it achieves adult size during adolescence[2] (**Fig. 1**). The anterior table is very thick (up to 12 mm), and the posterior table is thin (often < 1 mm). The frontal sinus outflow tract (FSOT) has an "hourglass" shape, with the narrowest portion being 1 to 3 mm in diameter (**Fig. 2**). Familiarity with the three-dimensional anatomy of the sinus and surrounding structures (orbital roof, anterior cranial fossa, FSOT, forehead/glabella) is critical to appropriate diagnosis and treatment of these injuries (**Fig. 3**).

Frontal sinus fractures account for 5% to 15% of traumatic maxillofacial injuries and are usually the result of high energy trauma.[3] Motor vehicle accidents and assaults account for the majority of these injuries.[3] Severe "through-and-through" injuries with violation of the anterior cranial fossa have trended downward with the introduction of seat belts and air bags.[3,4] Isolated anterior table fractures account for 33% of injuries, while combined anterior/posterior table and/or FSOT fractures account for 67% of fractures.[3] Isolated posterior table injuries are uncommon.

[a] Department of Otolaryngology –Head and Neck Surgery, University of California Davis, 2521 Stockton Boulevard, Suite 7200, Sacramento, CA 95817, USA; [b] Department of Otolaryngology-Head and Neck Surgery, University of Tennessee, 910 Madison Avenue, Suite 430, Memphis, TN 38103, USA
* Corresponding author.
E-mail address: ebstrong@ucdavis.edu

Facial Plast Surg Clin N Am 30 (2022) 71–83
https://doi.org/10.1016/j.fsc.2021.08.006

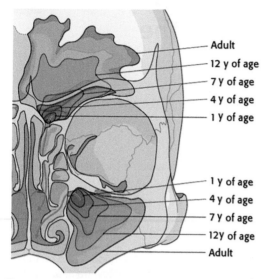

Adult
12 y of age
7 Y of age
4 y of age
1 Y of age

1 y of age
4 y of age
7 Y of age
12Y of age
Adult

Fig. 1. Frontal sinus development. The anterior ethmoid air cells invade the frontal bone at age 2. The sinus is fully developed by age 15. (*Reproduced with* permission from AO Surgery Reference, www. aosurgery.org (Copyright by AO Foundation, Switzerland).)

A thorough head and neck examination is essential with particular attention to the orbits, naso–orbito–ethmoid region, zygomaticomaxillary complex, and potential cerebrospinal fluid (CSF) leaks. Physical examination findings may include abrasions/lacerations, forehead contour irregularities, hematoma, tenderness, epistaxis, and clear rhinorrhea. Initial imaging should include fine-cut (∼1 mm) computed tomography (CT). 3D reconstructions are helpful for surgical planning when there is significant comminution or displacement of fracture fragments. If a CSF leak is suspected, a beta-2-transferrin assay should be obtained. It has excellent sensitivity (99%) and specificity (97%) but does take several days to process.[5]

TREATMENT ALGORITHM

Historically, frontal sinus fractures have been managed with large, open surgical approaches. The introduction of high-resolution CT and advanced transnasal endoscopic surgical techniques has ushered in a significant paradigm shift toward observation and minimally invasive treatment. An appropriate treatment strategy for frontal sinus fractures can be determined by evaluating the structural integrity of three anatomic parameters: (1) anterior table, (2) frontal sinus outflow tract, and (3) posterior table/dura. These findings can then be applied to the treatment algorithm presented in **Fig. 4**.

ANTERIOR TABLE FRACTURES

The authors divide these injuries into three groups (**Fig. 4**):
Mild: ≤4 mm displacement
Moderate: 4 to 6 mm displacement, moderate fracture area, with mild comminution
Severe: greater than 6 mm displacement, large fracture area with severe comminution

These anatomic parameters are used to select between 3 treatment strategies: observation, primary repair, and secondary camouflage. Surgical management is indicated when the risk of a contour deformity outweighs the risk of iatrogenic injury (ie, scaring, alopecia, paresthesia, etc).

Observation

Mucocele formation with isolated anterior table fractures is uncommon, and observation is appropriate for many of these injuries. The authors observe "mild" and less severe "moderate" fractures with close follow-up (see **Fig. 4**). A very small percentage may develop a contour deformity which can be corrected with a secondary camouflage procedure (see below). The goal of this approach is to avoid unnecessary surgery, while offering those few patients who need treatment a procedure that is equally efficacious to primary repair. The literature supports this conservative approach. In a series of 51 patients who underwent nonoperative management, Kim and colleagues[6] demonstrated that no patients with fracture displacement < 4 mm developed late forehead contour deformity at a mean follow-up of 18 months. Similarly, Dalla Torre and colleagues reported on 91 patients with fracture displacement ranging from 0 to 5 mm. Only 4 patients developed a frontal contour deformity, and none of the patients elected for secondary correction.[7]

Secondary Camouflage

The authors use secondary camouflage for patients found to have an esthetic deformity after observation or who present with an anterior table esthetic deformity. Secondary camouflage is very effective for patients with anterior table contour deformities that are completely healed.[8] The authors most often use an endoscopic brow lift approach; however, mid-forehead (through a rhytid or laceration) and upper blepharoplasty approaches can be equally effective.[9–15]

Endoscopic repair

A 3 to 5 cm parasagittal "working" incision is placed 3 cm posterior to the hairline and in line

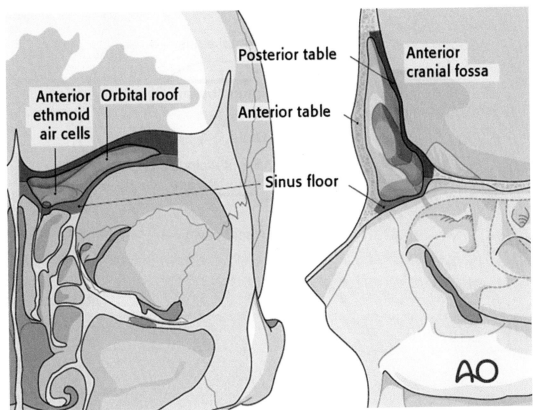

Fig. 2. Frontal sinus anatomy. The anterior table of the frontal sinus is thick bone and provides forehead contour. The posterior table is thinner and constitutes a portion of the anterior cranial fossa. The floor of the sinus makes up a portion of the orbital roof. The frontal sinus ostia is located in the medial, posterior, and inferior portion of the sinus floor. (*Reproduced with* permission from AO Surgery Reference, www.aosurgery.org (Copyright by AO Foundation, Switzerland).)

with the fracture (**Fig. 5**). A 1-2 cm "endoscope" incision is then placed at the same height, 6 cm medial to the working incision. Incisions may be moved toward the hairline for patients with receding hairlines. A subperiosteal dissection is performed with an endoscopic brow lift elevator. Dissection is performed without the endoscope and guided by palpation. Avoid tearing the periosteum, as it will help to maintain the optical cavity. After the deformity is exposed, a 4.0 mm 30-degree endoscope with rigid endosheath is inserted through the endoscope incision. A suture can be applied transcutaneously to tent the forehead skin/periosteum upward, optimizing the optical cavity (**Fig. 6**).

Porous polyethylene sheeting (0.85 mm) is used for reconstruction.[14–16] Titanium mesh should be avoided because the sharp edges make it very challenging to insert and manipulate. The implant is trimmed to cover the defect (**Fig. 7**). The implant is inserted through the working incision and manipulated over the defect using both internal instrumentation and external palpation (**Fig. 8**). The superior aspect of the implant is marked with a pen to maintain endoscopic orientation. The implant often needs to be modified after initial placement to optimize shape and contour. For deeper defects, it can be sutured in 2 to 3 layers forming an inverted pyramid (**Fig. 9**). Once the final implant is in place, a 25-gauge needle is passed through the skin and visualized endoscopically to determine optimal screw placement (ie, where multiple screws can be placed through a single incision). An 11 blade is used to make a 2 mm stab incision, and a 4-7 mm self-drilling screw is used to secure the screw through the implant at the periphery of the fracture (**Fig. 10**). Caution should be used to avoid losing screws as they pass through the soft tissue. Patient-specific implants also work very well (**Fig. 11**), avoiding the need for intraoperative contouring and reducing operative time. They are, however, significantly more expensive.

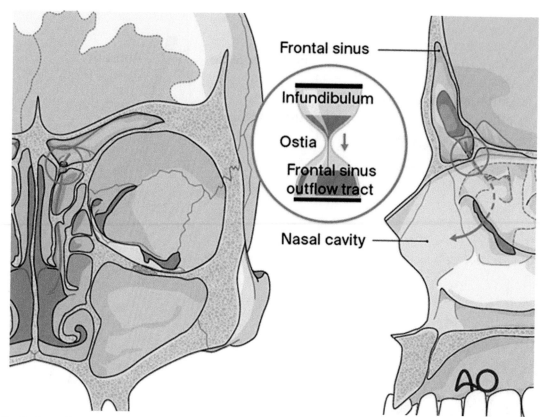

Fig. 3. Frontal sinus outflow tract. The frontal sinus outflow tract has an hourglass configuration with the infundibulum above and the frontal recess below. (*Reproduced with* permission from AO Surgery Reference, www. aosurgery.org (Copyright by AO Foundation, Switzerland).)

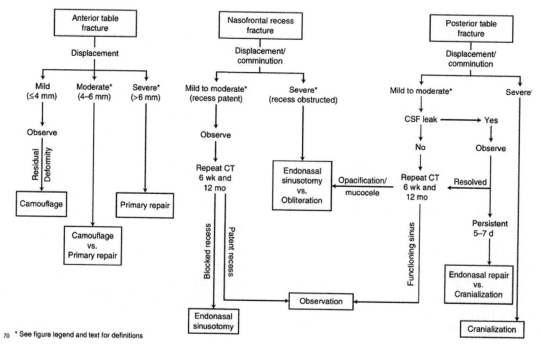

70 * See figure legend and text for definitions

Fig. 4. Treatment algorithm for frontal sinus fractures.

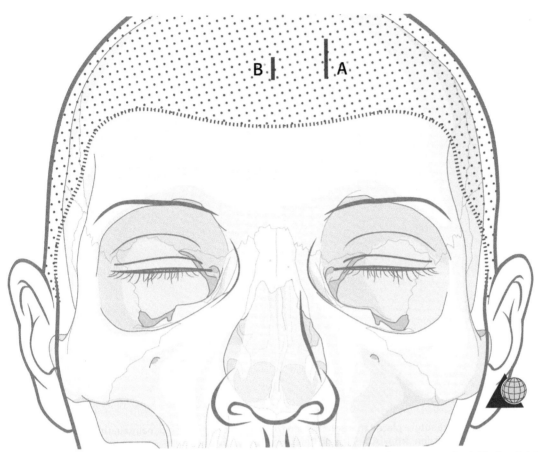

Fig. 5. Illustration demonstrating the incisions used for the endoscopic approach to an anterior table frontal sinus fracture. The "working incisions" (*A*) is placed directly above the fracture, while the "endoscope" incision (*B*) is placed approximately 6 cm medial. Both incisions are placed 3 cm above the hairline. (*Reproduced with* permission from AO Surgery Reference, www.aosurgery.org (Copyright by AO Foundation, Switzerland).)

Primary Repair

The authors treat more significant moderate and all severe fractures with primary repair (see **Fig. 4**). Primary repair can be performed via transcutaneous or transnasal endoscopic approaches. The authors prefer transcutaneous approaches when they can be performed through well-hidden incisions (ie, lacerations, rhytids, upper blepharoplasty). Transcutaneous approaches allow for direct visualization and bimanual manipulation, providing the best opportunity for an anatomic reduction. They are generally faster, require less equipment than transnasal approaches (Draf IIb or III), and avoid iatrogenic mucosal or skull base injury. However, both strategies will work, and the final decision is often based on the technical skills and experience of the surgeon.

Transcutaneous repair

A transcutaneous repair is used for patients with (1) lacerations providing direct access, (2) deep rhytids providing good camouflage for the incision, and (3) inferior fractures accessible via an upper blepharoplasty approach. These approaches have been used with good outcomes while avoiding the risks of a coronal incision.[13,17–19] Primary transcutaneous *endoscopic* repairs have been described (often combined with percutaneous screw placement), but success rates are variable.[9,10,15,20] A coronal incision is rarely used for an anterior table fractures and is reserved for injuries with severe comminution requiring direct visualization and manipulation of the bony segments.

Transnasal endoscopic repair

Transnasal endoscopic repairs have gained popularity in recent years.[3,21,22] Grayson and colleagues[23] published the largest case series demonstrating successful treatment of six anterior table fractures with an endoscopic Draf IIB or III. Other authors combined the endoscopic

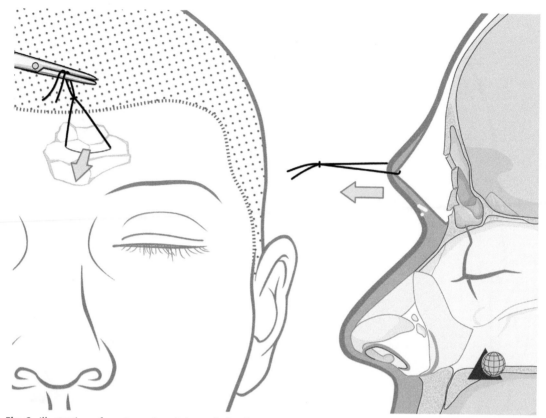

Fig. 6. Illustration of a suture placed through the skin to apply traction and help maintain the optical cavity. (*Reproduced with* permission from AO Surgery Reference, www.aosurgery.org (Copyright by AO Foundation, Switzerland).)

approach with a transcutaneous trephination for far lateral fractures where endoscopic instrumentation is difficult.[24,25] They describe the use of bone hooks, elevators, and even foley catheter balloons. The primary risk of a balloon catheter is the lack of tactile feedback when applying pressure to the thin posterior table bone. The surgeon will not be aware of a posterior table injury until he/she visualizes a posterior table fracture and sees a CSF leak.

FRONTAL SINUS OUTFLOW TRACT FRACTURES

Significant FSOT injury can lead to chronic sinusitis, mucocele/mucopyocele formation, and osteomyelitis.[3,26] Historically, surgical management focused on aggressive open approaches (ie, obliteration or cranialization) to avoid long-term sequelae. Unfortunately, complication rates for these techniques range from 10% to 17%.[27] This must be weighed against the risks of a more conservative observational approach in less severe injuries. Current high-resolution CT scanners provide outstanding bony resolution, allowing

surgeons to more accurately identify FSOT injuries. Additionally, endoscopic evaluation can be used to complement CT.[23] Despite these tools, some controversy remains over what constitutes a "significant" (ie, operative) FSOT injury.[28]

The authors use high-resolution CT to separate FSOT injuries into two major categories (see **Fig. 4**):

Mild to moderate (injuries ranging from nondisplaced to moderately displaced fractures narrowing the outflow tract without complete obstruction of the lumen)

Severe (complete collapse of the frontal sinus outflow tract) (**Fig. 12**).

These anatomic parameters are used to select between 3 treatment strategies: (1) observation with medical management, (2) endoscopic frontal sinusotomy, and (3) primary repair.

Observation with Medical Management

Medical management includes topical nasal steroids at 1 week and sinus irrigations at 3 weeks

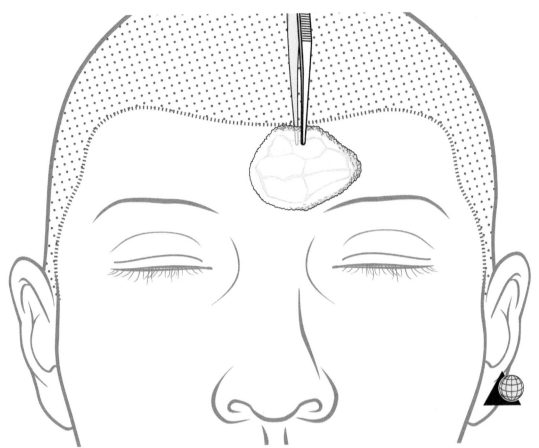

Fig. 7. A 85-mm-thick sheet of porous polyethylene sheeting is placed on the skin over the defect and used as a template to approximate the size of the implant to be used. (*Reproduced with* permission from AO Surgery Reference, www.aosurgery.org (Copyright by AO Foundation, Switzerland).)

after the initial injury. Follow-up CT scans are performed at 6 weeks and 12 months to assess frontal sinus aeration. Patients with mild mucosal edema may continue medical management. Mucosal edema will clear in many patients and no surgical intervention will be required. This has been demonstrated in several small case series.[29,30] Sinus opacification or mucocele formation will require an endoscopic frontal sinusotomy, which has been referred to as a "frontal sinus rescue procedure" (see below).

Frontal Sinus Rescue Procedure (Endoscopic Frontal Sinusotomy)

Patients who are observed may have recurrent sinusitis, sinus opacification, or delayed mucocele formation. These patients will require surgical treatment with an endoscopic frontal sinusotomy (Draf IIb or III).[31] Although it may be counterintuitive, a Draf procedure performed for a frontal mucocele is often easier to accomplish than when performed for inflammatory disease. This is

because mucoceles usually expand toward the nasal cavity, widening the drainage pathway, resulting in less drilling close to vital structures. Reliable patient follow up is required for this approach.

Surgical technique

Understanding the anatomy of the anterior sinonasal cavity is essential for a safe endoscopic frontal sinusotomy (**Fig. 13**A).[32] An endoscopic anterior ethmoidectomy is performed, skeletonizing the anterior skull base and lamina papyracea. Angled endoscopes (30, 45, or 70°) and cutting instrumentation are used to remove the entire Agger nasi cell, allowing visualization of the FSOT. A 2 × 2 cm anterior septectomy is performed to allow visualization/access across the midline (see **Fig. 13**B). The head of the middle turbinate marks the posterior boundary of the septectomy. The inferior limit is identified once the upper half of the contralateral middle turbinate is visualized. Next, the skull base mucosa anterior

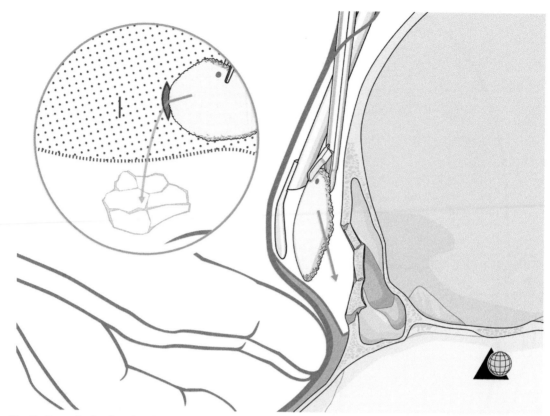

Fig. 8. Once the implant has been trimmed to size, the superior edge is marked to maintain orientation after insertion. The implant is then inserted through the working incision under direct visualization with the endoscope. (*Reproduced with* permission from AO Surgery Reference, www.aosurgery.org (Copyright by AO Foundation, Switzerland).)

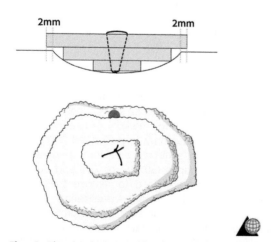

Fig. 9. The implant may be layered and sutured together for greater stability in deeper defects. (*Reproduced with* permission from AO Surgery Reference, www.aosurgery.org (Copyright by AO Foundation, Switzerland).)

to the olfactory groove is elevated posteriorly until encountering the first olfactory neuron which marks the posterior limit of the dissection. A high-speed angled 4 mm diamond burr is used to remove the floor of the frontal sinus (see **Fig. 13**C). Drilling is initiated laterally, removing the bone of the middle turbinate axilla and frontal process of the maxilla until encountering (but not violating) the periosteum under the nasal skin (see **Fig. 13**D). The frontal beak and intersinus septum are drilled down to create a common, horseshoe shaped, midline drainage pathway for the frontal sinuses (see **Fig. 13**E). Exposed bone over the frontal beak can be grafted with septal mucosa harvested from the superior septectomy window,[33] dressed with silastic sheeting, or left alone to remucosalize.

Primary Repair

Acute endoscopic fracture repair

Endoscopic frontal sinusotomy for sinusitis and mucocele is described earlier (see *frontal sinus rescue procedure – surgical technique*). The

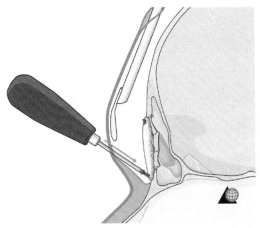

Fig. 10. A self-drilling screw is passed through the edge of the implant and into stable bone. (*Reproduced with* permission from AO Surgery Reference, www.aosurgery.org (Copyright by AO Foundation, Switzerland).)

same surgical technique can be used for management of acute FSOT injuries. However, the surgeon must be aware that the frontal process of the maxilla and frontal bone will be mobile and the endonasal anatomy will be distorted, increasing the risk of iatrogenic injury. It will be necessary to drill and possibly remove mobile bone fragments to obtain adequate visualization into the frontal sinus. The acute angulation requires use of a 70° endoscope, angled drills, and frontal sinus instrumentation. A unilateral (Draf IIb) or bilateral (Draf III) can be used depending on the location of the injury; however, visualization can be challenging and the Draf III approach will provide the largest optical cavity and working area.

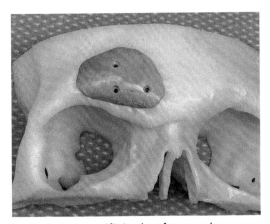

Fig. 11. Patient-specific implant for secondary camouflage. These implants can be placed through an endoscopic brow or open approach.

Once the FSOT is open, the integrity of the posterior table is assessed (See **Fig. 4**). Maintenance of the outflow tract postoperatively is critical. The authors use mucosal grafts when possible (obtained from nasal floor) to line the new FSOT. The grafts are held in place with rolled 0.4 mm silastic sheeting and bolstered by Posisep (Hemostasis LLC, St. Paul, MN) nasal packing. Finger cot stents or silastic sheets are often placed in the middle meatus to reduce the risk of scaring. Stent and packing are removed at 3 weeks. Multiple authors have described similar techniques, but long-term outcome studies are not yet available.[23,34–36]

Obliteration

Frontal sinus obliteration is an open technique performed via a coronal incision. A frontal sinusotomy and meticulous removal of all frontal sinus mucosa is critical followed by obstruction of the FSOT with fascia and bone grafts. The sinus cavity is then obliterated with autologous material (ie, fat, fascia lata, pericranium). The surgical technique is described elsewhere and is beyond the scope of this article.[26,28,37] Although traditionally considered the "gold standard" treatment for complex frontal sinus fractures, long-term mucocele formation is a significant risk. The actual incidence is unknown because mucoceles may occur 10 to 20 years after the procedure.[38] In the largest frontal sinus fracture cohort study to date (n = 857), Rodriguez and colleagues[28] demonstrated that among the 504 patients who underwent surgical management, 61 patients developed complications (7.1%). Sixty of those 61 cases involved FSOT obstruction. This highlights why obliteration is being reevaluated and more conservative endoscopic techniques are gaining traction. The authors have not performed sinus obliteration since adopting the current algorithm (see **Fig. 4**).

POSTERIOR TABLE FRACTURES

Historically, posterior table fractures were routinely managed with cranialization. Given that complication rates ranging from 10% to 17%,[27] recent trends have moved toward conservative management. In a retrospective cohort by Choi and colleagues[39], 46 posterior table fractures (including six with CSF leak and 16 with comminution and or displacement) were treated with observation, and all had resolution of CSF leak and lack of any complications at a mean follow-up of 1 year. Although the results must be interpreted with caution (ie, retrospective cohort design and limited follow up) follow-up, and so forth), the authors have had a similar clinical experience.

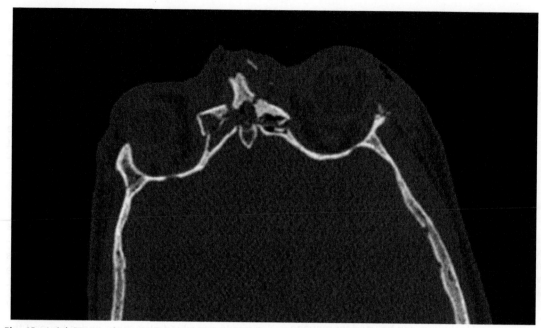

Fig. 12. Axial CT scan demonstrating a severe frontal sinus outflow tract fracture.

The authors use CT imaging and endoscopy to group these injuries into two major categories based on the degree of displacement/comminution of the posterior table and the presence of a CSF leak (see **Fig. 4**):

Mild-to-moderate injuries include fractures ranging from nondisplaced up to 4 mm of displacement, mild pneumocephalus, and mild to moderate posterior table comminution.

Severe injuries include fractures with greater than 4 mm of displacement, involving large areas of the posterior table, severe pneumocephalus, dural disruption with persistent CSF rhinorrhea, and severe comminution.

These anatomic parameters are used to select between 3 treatment strategies: (1) observation and medical management, (2) endonasal sinusotomy, and (3) cranialization.

Observation and Medical Management

Mild-to-moderate injuries are treated with close observation for CSF leak and supportive medical management. If a leak is present, the patient is kept at bed rest with CSF leak precautions for 1 week. Most leaks will resolve.[40–42] If the leak persists, an endonasal sinusotomy is performed and the leak is repaired endoscopically (see endonasal sinusotomy and CSF leak repair). If the leak resolves, medical management includes topical nasal steroids at 1 week and sinus irrigations at 3 weeks after resolution of the leak. Follow-up CT scans are performed at 6 weeks and 12 months to assess frontal sinus aeration. Patients with mild mucosal edema may continue medical management. Mucosal edema will clear in many patients and no surgical intervention will be required. If there is progression of inflammatory disease (sinus opacification or mucocele formation), a transnasal endoscopic sinusotomy is performed (see "frontal sinus rescue procedure – surgical technique").

Endonasal sinusotomy and CSF leak repair

This technique involves a Draf III approach to the FSOT as described earlier (see "acute endoscopic fracture repair"). Once a Draf III is completed, most leaks are visible with a 45° or 70° endoscope. Fluorescein can be used but is not typically necessary. Far lateral leaks may require secondary access via an upper eyelid blepharoplasty incision. Endoscopic orbital decompression techniques for "far lateral" frontal sinus access have been described.[43] However, the current authors feel that there is less risk to the orbit with an upper blepharoplasty incision than orbital decompression.

Once the defect is visualized, the surrounding mucosa is circumferentially removed to clearly identify the leak. Telescoped bony segments are either reduced or removed depending on the severity of injury. Although other authors have described the use of radiofrequency devices to

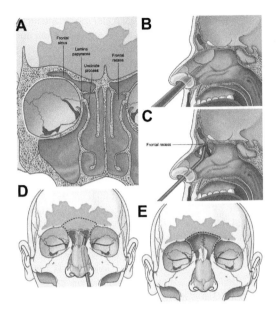

Fig. 13. (*A*) Coronal illustration of the anterior ethmoid sinuses, frontal sinus, and anterior skull base. (*B*) Illustration of an anterior septectomy used to visualize the anterior skull base bilaterally. (*C*) Illustration of a high-speed diamond bur being used to remove the floor of the frontal sinus. (*D*) Illustration of a high-speed diamond bur being used to remove the frontal process of the maxilla, identifying the periosteum of the overlying skin. (*E*) Illustration of completed frontal sinusotomy with the entire frontal sinus floor removed, forming a single common drainage pathway into the nose. (*Reprinted with permission from Shaye DA, & Strong EB. (2020). Frontal Bone and Frontal Sinus Injuries. Elsevier*[32])

remove frontal sinus mucosa,[23] the current authors treat frontal sinus CSF leaks in the same fashion as ethmoid and sphenoid skull base leaks and have not found this necessary. After complete

exposure, dural substitutes, that is, Duragen® (Integra, Plainsboro, NJ) or Biodesign® (Cook Medical, Bloomington, IN), are used as underlay grafts for defects larger than 5 mm. Free mucosal overlay grafts are then used to cover the defect. Nasoseptal flaps are rarely used because they will often not reach for enough to cover the injured area. Tissue glue is often used to maintain the mucosal positioning, and absorbable packing (surgicell, gel foam, posisep) is placed to fill the remainder of the sinus to maintain the graft position. Finally, 0.4 mm silastic sheeting is trimmed, placed in the FSOT to minimize postop narrowing, and maintained in place with absorbable packing (posisep). The packing is left in place for 3 weeks.

Grayson and colleagues[44] have published the largest series describing this technique. They performed endoscopic endonasal approach to posterior table frontal sinus fractures with active CSF leak in 41 patients, with 100% success rate at a mean follow-up of 26 months.[23,34] Fracture sizes were on average 17.1 × 9.1 mm and repaired with overlay grafts or nasoseptal flap alone or with the addition of a porcine small intestine submucosal underlay graft when there was a bony gap greater than 5 mm.

Cranialization

Severe fractures (**Fig. 14**) are usually not amenable to endoscopic repair and are treated with cranialization. A combined neurosurgical and craniomaxillofacial approach is usually necessary. The procedure can often be performed directly through the sinus; however, more extensive injuries may require a formal craniotomy. It is critical to maintain the integrity of the pericranial flap for dural

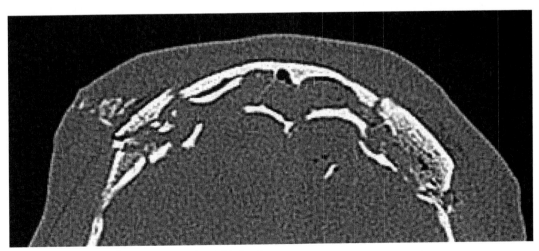

Fig. 14. Axial CT scan of a severe posterior table fracture.

repair. The surgical technique is described elsewhere and is beyond the scope of this article.[45]

SUMMARY

Although open surgical repair has been the "gold standard" for management of frontal sinus fractures, advances in CT imaging and endoscopic surgical techniques have revolutionized the approach to these injuries. More conservative treatments including observation with medical management, secondary camouflage, and endonasal sinusotomy continue to gain traction in the literature. Long-term follow-up of more complex injuries remains critical.

CLINICS CARE POINTS

- Isolated anterior table fractures with ≤4 mm of displacement are unlikely to require surgical intervention.

- Many isolated anterior table fractures between 4 to 6 mm may be observed. This approach avoids unnecessary surgery, while using minimally invasive techniques (as efficacious as primary repair) to camouflage the few esthetic deformities that occur.

- Recent evidence supports a conservative approach for mild/moderately displaced frontal sinus outflow tract (FSOT) injuries, as a vast majority of these will maintain clinic patency. A frontal sinus rescue procedure (Draf IIb/III) can be used for those sinuses that obstruct after observation.

- Mildly displaced posterior table fractures can be safely observed with close clinical follow-up.

- More severe FSOT and posterior table injuries can be managed acutely with endoscopic technique by surgeons with extensive endoscopic skull base experience.

DISCLOSURES

The authors have nothing to disclose.

REFERENCES

1. Le P, Martinez R, Black J. Frontal sinus fracture management meta-analysis: endoscopic versus open repair. J Craniofac Surg 2020.
2. Anon JB, Rontal M, Zinreich SJ. Anatomy of the paransasal sinuses. New York: Thieme; 1996.
3. Strong EB, Pahlavan N, Saito D. Frontal sinus fractures: a 28-year retrospective review. Otolaryngol Head Neck Surg 2006;135:774–9.
4. Weathers WM, Wolfswinkel EM, Hatef DA, et al. Frontal sinus fractures: a conservative shift. Craniomaxillofac Trauma Reconstr 2013;6:155–60.
5. Meco C, Oberascher G, Arrer E, et al. Beta-trace protein test: new guidelines for the reliable diagnosis of cerebrospinal fluid fistula. Otolaryngol Head Neck Surg 2003;129:508–17.
6. Kim DW, Yoon ES, Lee BI, et al. Fracture depth and delayed contour deformity in frontal sinus anterior wall fracture. J Craniofac Surg 2012;23:991–4.
7. Dalla Torre D, Burtscher D, Kloss-Brandstatter A, et al. Management of frontal sinus fractures–treatment decision based on metric dislocation extent. J Craniomaxillofac Surg 2014;42:1515–9.
8. Dedhia RD, Morisada MV, Tollefson TT, et al. Contemporary management of frontal sinus fractures. Curr Opin Otolaryngol Head Neck Surg 2019;27:253–60.
9. Graham HD 3rd, Spring P. Endoscopic repair of frontal sinus fracture: case report. J Craniomaxillofac Trauma 1996;2:52–5.
10. Strong EB, Kellman RM. Endoscopic repair of anterior table–frontal sinus fractures. Facial Plast Surg Clin North Am 2006;14:25–9.
11. Lappert PW, Lee JW. Treatment of an isolated outer table frontal sinus fracture using endoscopic reduction and fixation. Plast Reconstr Surg 1998;102:1642–5.
12. De Cordier BC, de la Torre JI, Al-Hakeem MS, et al. Endoscopic forehead lift: review of technique, cases, and complications. Plast Reconstr Surg 2002;110:1558–68 [discussion 1569–70].
13. Kinzinger M, Steele TO, Chin O, et al. Degree of frontal bone exposure via upper blepharoplasty incision: considerations for frontal sinus fracture. Otolaryngol Head Neck Surg 2019;160:468–71.
14. Arcuri F, Baragiotta N, Poglio G, et al. Post-traumatic deformity of the anterior frontal table managed by the placement of a titanium mesh via an endoscopic approach. Br J Oral Maxillofac Surg 2012;50:e53–4.
15. Kim KK, Mueller R, Huang F, et al. Endoscopic repair of anterior table: frontal sinus fractures with a Medpor implant. Otolaryngol Head Neck Surg 2007;136:568–72.
16. Strong EB. Endoscopic repair of anterior table frontal sinus fractures. Facial Plast Surg 2009;25:43–8.
17. Kim J, Choi H. A review of subbrow approach in the management of non-complicated anterior table frontal sinus fracture. Arch Craniofac Surg 2016;17:186–9.
18. Hahn HM, Lee YJ, Park MC, et al. Reduction of closed frontal sinus fractures through suprabrow approach. Arch Craniofac Surg 2017;18:230–7.
19. Alinasab B, Fridman-Bengtsson O, Sunnergren O, et al. The supratarsal approach for correction of

anterior frontal bone fractures. J Craniofac Surg 2018;29:1906–9.

20. Strong EB, Buchalter GM, Moulthrop TH. Endoscopic repair of isolated anterior table frontal sinus fractures. Arch Facial Plast Surg 2003;5:514–21.

21. Guy WM, Brissett AE. Contemporary management of traumatic fractures of the frontal sinus. Otolaryngol Clin North Am 2013;46:733–48.

22. Shumrick KA. Endoscopic management of frontal sinus fractures. Otolaryngol Clin North Am 2007;40: 329–36.

23. Grayson JW, Jeyarajan H, Illing EA, et al. Changing the surgical dogma in frontal sinus trauma: transnasal endoscopic repair. Int Forum Allergy Rhinol 2017;7:441–9.

24. Steiger JD, Chiu AG, Francis DO, et al. Endoscopic-assisted reduction of anterior table frontal sinus fractures. Laryngoscope 2006;116:1978–81.

25. Jin HR, Shim WS, Jung HJ. Minimally invasive technique to reduce the isolated anterior wall fracture of the frontal sinus. J Craniofac Surg 2019;30:2375–7.

26. Wallis A, Donald PJ. Frontal sinus fractures: a review of 72 cases. Laryngoscope 1988;98:593–8.

27. Adelson RT, Wei C, Palmer JN. Frontal sinus fractures. In: Palmer JN, Chiu AG, Adappa ND, editors. Atlas of endoscopic and sinonasal skull base surgery. Philadelphia: Elsevier; 2013. p. 337–56.

28. Rodriguez ED, Stanwix MG, Nam AJ, et al. Twenty-six-year experience treating frontal sinus fractures: a novel algorithm based on anatomical fracture pattern and failure of conventional techniques. Plast Reconstr Surg 2008;122:1850–66.

29. Smith TL, Han JK, Loehrl TA, et al. Endoscopic management of the frontal recess in frontal sinus fractures: a shift in the paradigm? Laryngoscope 2002; 112:784–90.

30. Jafari A, Nuyen BA, Salinas CR, et al. Spontaneous ventilation of the frontal sinus after fractures involving the frontal recess. Am J Otol 2015;36: 837–42.

31. Weber R, Draf W, Kratzsch B, et al. Modern concepts of frontal sinus surgery. Laryngoscope 2001; 111:137–46.

32. Shaye DA, Strong EB. Frontal bone and frontal sinus injuries. In: Dorafshar AH, Rodriguez E, Manson PN, editors. Facial trauma surgery. New York: Elsevier; 2020. p. 88–105.

33. Illing EA, Woodworth BA. Management of frontal sinus cerebrospinal fluid leaks and encephaloceles. Otolaryngol Clin North Am 2016;49:1035–50.

34. Banks C, Grayson J, Cho DY, et al. Frontal sinus fractures and cerebrospinal fluid leaks: a change in surgical paradigm. Curr Opin Otolaryngol Head Neck Surg 2020;28:52–60.

35. Choi KJ, Chang B, Woodard CR, et al. Survey of current practice patterns in the management of frontal sinus fractures. Craniomaxillofac Trauma Reconstr 2017;10:106–16.

36. Elkahwagi M, Eldegwi A. What is the role of the endoscope in the sinus preservation management of frontal sinus fractures? J Oral Maxillofac Surg 2020;78:1811.e1–9.

37. Rohrich RJ, Hollier LH. Management of frontal sinus fractures. Changing concepts. Clin Plast Surg 1992; 19:219–32.

38. Hansen FS, van der Poel NA, Freling NJM, et al. Mucocele formation after frontal sinus obliteration. Rhinology 2018;56:106–10.

39. Choi M, Li Y, Shapiro SA, et al. A 10-year review of frontal sinus fractures: clinical outcomes of conservative management of posterior table fractures. Plast Reconstr Surg 2012;130:399–406.

40. Mincy JE. Posttraumatic cerebrospinal fluid fistula of the frontal fossa. J Trauma 1966;6:618–22.

41. Bell RB, Dierks EJ, Homer L, et al. Management of cerebrospinal fluid leak associated with craniomaxillofacial trauma. J Oral Maxillofac Surg 2004;62: 676–84.

42. Brodie HA, Thompson TC. Management of complications from 820 temporal bone fractures. Am J Otol 1997;18:188–97.

43. Poczos P, Kurbanov A, Keller JT, et al. Medial and superior orbital decompression: improving access for endonasal endoscopic frontal sinus surgery. Ann Otol Rhinol Laryngol 2015;124:987–95.

44. Grayson J.W., Jeyarajan H., Illing E.A., et al. Changing the surgical dogma in frontal sinus trauma: transnasal endoscopic repair. Available at: https://onlinelibrary.wiley.com/doi/full/10.1002/alr.21897?casa_token=k6nEPLi3XS8AAAAA%3ATmHmvepPTehmfQE-MAjt5kukClydUOIYBrFqvepYLlxZIB_STORvFK2d0KCEuciS6_ksnFvZJ5S2_3FU.

45. Strong EB, Shaye DA, Steele TO, et al. Frontal sinus fractures: a surgical management paradigm. Otorinolaringologia 2017;67:10–25.

Mandibular Condylar Fractures

Sean Mooney, MD[a], Rahul D. Gulati, MD[a], Steve Yusupov, DDS, MD[b], Sydney C. Butts, MD[c],*

KEYWORDS

- Condylar fracture • Maxillo-mandibular fixation • Malocclusion • Internal fixation
- Retromandibular approach

KEY POINTS

- The condyle is a frequently fractured subsite of the mandible and the most frequently injured in children
- Standard outcomes measures should be recorded for all patients including opening, protrusion, lateral excursion, occlusion, chin deviation with opening, facial symmetry, pain, and TMJ derangement
- Patients with fractures with significant displacement, dislocation, or override with ramus shortening have the poorest prognosis for functional restoration when treated closed. These patients may best be served with open treatment
- Children younger than 12 years, even with displaced or dislocated fractures, have good functional outcomes with closed treatment

INTRODUCTION

The mandibular condyle is estimated to be involved in 25% to 45% of adult mandibular fractures. Up to 52% of mandibular fractures involve the condyle in the pediatric population.[1–3] Most individuals sustaining condylar fractures are men and young, with average ages between 20 and 40 years, and an estimated 40% to 50% have a second fracture elsewhere in the mandible, often a contralateral parasymphyseal or body fracture.[4–6] Bilateral condylar fractures may occur.[2,3] Fractures of the condyle may result from a direct blow to the condylar region or to another region of the mandible with the force transmitted to this weak area.[7] Common causes of mandibular fractures include assault, motor vehicle accidents or falls, especially onto the chin as can occur during skateboarding and bicycle riding.[8]

ANATOMY AND FRACTURE CLASSIFICATION

The condyle has 3 subsites: the condylar head, the condylar neck, and the subcondylar area.[9,10] (**Fig. 1**) The condylar head is broad and rounded articulating in the glenoid fossa and completely surrounded by the temporomandibular joint (TMJ) capsule (**Fig. 2**). At the inferior portion of the TMJ capsule, the condyle tapers to the region of the condylar neck and then widens at its attachment to the mandible forming the condylar base or subcondylar region.[11]

The TMJ functions as both a hinge and sliding joint, also known as ginglymoarthrodial, and is capable of opening, closing, left and right excursion, jaw protrusion, and retrotrusion.[12] Left and right lateral excursion occur, by the pterygoid muscles pulling the mandible toward the contralateral side (ie, contraction of the right medial and

Disclosure: The authors have nothing to disclose.
[a] Department of Otolaryngology, SUNY Downstate Health Sciences University, 450 Clarkson Avenue, Box 126, Brooklyn, NY 11203, USA; [b] Staten Island University Hospital/Northwell Health, 256-C Mason Avenue, Staten Island, NY 10305, USA; [c] Division of Facial Plastic and Reconstructive Surgery, Department of Otolaryngology, SUNY Downstate Health Sciences University, Kings County Hospital Center, 450 Clarkson Avenue, Box 126, Brooklyn, NY 11203, USA
* Corresponding author.
E-mail address: sydney.butts@downstate.edu

Facial Plast Surg Clin N Am 30 (2022) 85–98
https://doi.org/10.1016/j.fsc.2021.08.007
1064-7406/22/© 2021 Elsevier Inc. All rights reserved.

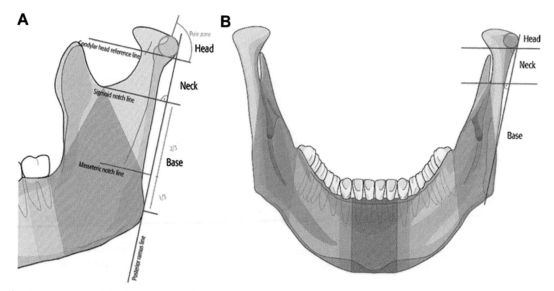

Fig. 1. AOCMF condylar fracture classification system. (A) saggital view; (B) posterior view. (*From* Neff A, Cornelius C-P, Rasse M, Torre D, Audigé L. The comprehensive AOCMF classification system: condylar process fractures-level 3 tutorial. *Craniomaxillofacial trauma & reconstruction.* 2014;7(1_suppl):44-58.; with permission.)

lateral pterygoid muscles causes lateral excursion to the left; see **Fig. 2**).[12,13]

Classification of condylar fractures should allow for clear communication among specialists and consist of an adequate number of domains to describe the fracture in several dimensions.[14,15]

The terminology used in these systems warrants review. The terms "displacement" and "dislocation" have different meanings in European medical journals compared to those from Great Britain and North America.[10,11,15] The definition that will be used in this article for fracture "displacement" is the relationship of the caudal end of the condyle relative to the mandibular ramus. There may be no displacement, minimal tilting, or medial or lateral displacement resulting in overlap of the segments.[9,10] Displacement can be quantified as the degrees of angulation of the bones at the fracture site and millimeters of overlap between the condylar segment and the ramus.[10,16] The term "dislocation" refers to the location of the condylar head relative to the glenoid fossa. The term "intracapsular" has been used in reports to refer to fractures of the condylar head which is surrounded by the TMJ capsule but recently the term "diacapitular" was proposed to describe this fracture that may extend beyond the capsule.[10,16,17]

Lindahl's (*1977*) system of condylar fractures includes 3 domains: fracture level, displacement, and condylar dislocation[9,18,19] (**Fig. 3**). Loukota and colleagues (*2005*) introduced a system that was adopted by the Strasbourg Osteosynthesis Research Group (SORG) that distinguished

condylar subsites defining the demarcation between the condylar neck and the subcondylar region using "Line A" a horizontal line drawn tangent to the deepest part of the sigmoid notch and perpendicular to a vertical line parallel to the posterior border of the mandibular ramus (**Fig. 4**).[16] Condylar neck fractures result from a fracture line wherein more than 50% of the length is above line A, whereas subcondylar fractures are generated by fracture lines 50% or more of whose length is below line A (see **Fig. 4**).

In 2014, the AOCMF published a classification system that includes reproducible landmarks that demarcate fracture levels similar to Loukota's system (see **Fig. 1**).[11] Angulation/displacement and dislocation of the condylar segment is similar conceptually to Lindahl's system. This system allows for coding of the specific fractures and we refer the reader to this article for a review of all the domains.[11]

The need for consensus on the use of classification systems was the focus of a study by McLeod et al who reviewed 88 articles published between 2016 and 2019 and identified which condylar fracture classification systems were used. Forty papers used a previously published classification system (*the top three cited were Loukota 2005 = 12; Lindahl 1977 = 10; Neff 2014 = 9*).[9,11,16] Thirty-one published studies did not use a fracture classification system and 17 studies included a system not previously published.[14] McLeod concluded with a call for consistency in terminology and classification of condylar fractures and for peer reviewers

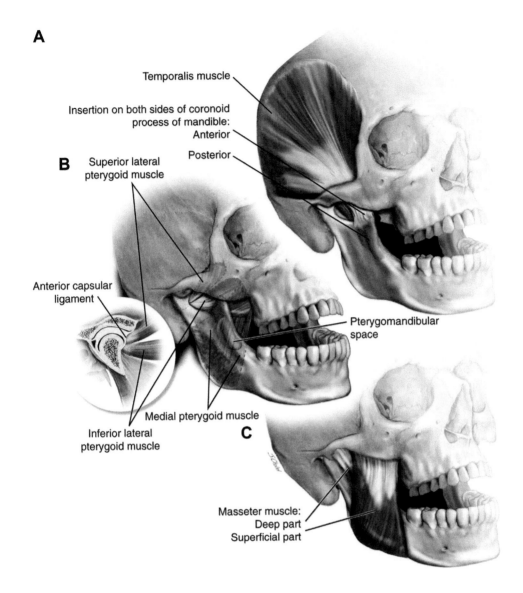

A

Temporalis muscle

Insertion on both sides of coronoid
process of mandible:
Anterior

B   Superior lateral
pterygoid muscle

Posterior

Anterior capsular
ligament

Pterygomandibular
space

Medial pterygoid muscle

Inferior lateral
pterygoid muscle   C

Masseter muscle:
Deep part
Superficial part

Fig. 2. Muscles of mastication. (*From* Morris, C. The anatomy of the face mouth and jaws. In: Kademani D, Tiwana PS, editors. Atlas of oral and maxillofacial surgery. St Louis (MO): Saunders; 2016.; with permission.)

and journal editors considering studies for publication to encourage more rigor in this area.[14]

CLINICAL PRESENTATION

The initial assessment of all craniofacial trauma begins with the primary trauma survey and emergency management of any potentially life-threatening injuries. Mandibular fractures can result in airway compromise secondary to floor of mouth swelling, hematoma or secondary to posterior displacement of the tongue. Displaced fractures of the mandibular condyle may result in a limited mouth opening, making specialized airway

management devices such as the video laryngoscope or flexible fiber-optic bronchoscope necessary for endotracheal intubation.[20] Identification of cervical spine injuries during the initial trauma survey is critical, and the incidence of concomitant cervical spine injuries in patients with mandibular fractures has been reported at 1% to 7%.[21]

On examination, patients with condylar fractures may have tenderness and edema of the pre-auricular area; chin lacerations, ecchymosis, or edema; malocclusion, trismus, and deviation of the chin with opening.[12,22] Displaced unilateral condylar fractures can result in a loss of vertical ramus height, premature contact of the molar

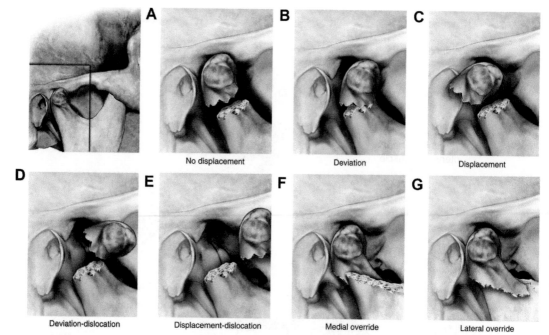

Fig. 3. Lindahl classification of condylar fractures. (*From* Reddy, L., Bishonp, C.M. Mandibular Condyle Fractures. In: Kademani D, Tiwana PS, editors. Atlas of oral and maxillofacial surgery. St Louis (MO): Saunders; 2016; with permission.)

teeth on the injured side, and a posterior open bite on the contralateral side (**Fig. 5**). The chin can deviate toward the side of injury during opening due to unopposed contralateral lateral pterygoid muscle contraction.[23] Patients with bilateral condylar fractures have bilateral ramus height shortening and premature molar contact resulting in an anterior open bite malocclusion. Trismus, defined as a maximal incisal opening less than 40 mm, may be present due to functional interferences of the fracture segments, joint hemarthrosis, or pain.[12,22] Care must be taken in evaluating pediatric patients with a low threshold for imaging

with CT scan—especially children presenting after a fall on the chin—to avoid missing a fracture.[3]

IMAGING

Helical computed tomography is the gold standard for radiographic diagnosis and can be reconstructed into 3-dimensional images.[7] The mandible series is a set of plain x-rays taken from 5 different views (**Fig. 6**). Towne's view (patient has their head angled downward 30°), lateral oblique, and lateral views are best for visualizing the condyle. Panoramic orthopantomogram may

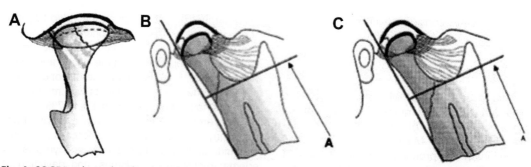

Fig. 4. SOGR/Loukota classification of condylar fractures. (*A*) Condylar head fracture, (*B*) condylar neck fracture, and (*C*) subcondylar fracture. (*From* Loukota R, Eckelt U, De Bont L, Rasse M. Subclassification of fractures of the condylar process of the mandible. *British journal of oral and maxillofacial surgery.* 2005;43(1):72-73.; with permission.)

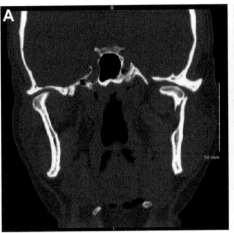
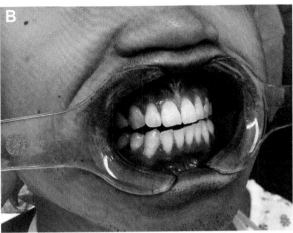

Fig. 5. Patient with left condylar neck fracture, medial displacement/override (*A*) and right posterior open bite (*B*).

also be obtained and provides a single composite panoramic image.[24]

GOALS OF TREATMENT/TREATMENT DECISION MAKING

Unlike other areas of the mandible, restoration of the condylar segment to its preinjury position is not required for the function to be restored. The following are the 5 outcomes that should be measured to assess attainment of treatment goals:

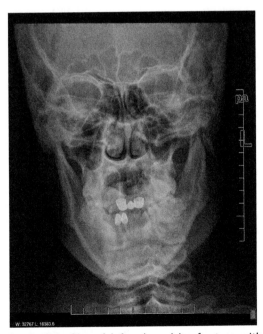

Fig. 6. Plain film of left subcondylar fracture with lateral override.

(1) pain-free mouth opening, with an interincisal opening of 40 mm or more; (2) full movement of the jaw in all excursions with no deviation on opening; (3) restoration of preinjury occlusion; (4) avoidance of TMJ dysfunction; and (5) facial and jaw symmetry.[25] There are 3 main treatment options offered to patients. Closed treatment includes 2 possibilities: a conservative therapy regimen of analgesics, soft diet and jaw mobility exercises or maxillomandibular fixation (MMF) to either completely immobilize the mandible or allow limited guided movement controlled by elastics attached to arch bars or MMF screws (**Fig. 7**). It is important to recognize that closed treatment is not equivalent to closed reduction.[17,26] In nondisplaced fractures, the condylar segment may assume a normal or near-normal position. Fracture segments that are displaced or dislocated may reside in a nonanatomical position even after a period of MMF, yet the patient can achieve normal occlusion and jaw movements at the completion of treatment (**Fig. 8**).[26] One stated advantage of open reduction and internal fixation is alignment and stability of the condylar segment, which is thought to provide the best chance for full functional rehabilitation.[26]

Survey studies that assess practice patterns provide a snapshot of surgeon preferences at a given period and provide an understanding of the evolution of condylar fracture management over time. In 1998, Baker and colleagues surveyed selected expert oral maxillofacial surgeons regarding the management of different presentations of condylar fractures. Among respondents, open reduction, internal fixation (ORIF) of the condylar fracture was most often chosen in the scenarios when the condylar process was

Class I Elastics   ## Class II Elastics   ## Class III Elastics

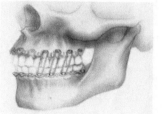

Vector:	• Neutral	• Anterosuperior force vector to mandible	• Posterosuperior force vector to mandible
Orthodontic indication:	• Class I malocclusion	• Class II malocclusion	• Class III malocclusion
Protocol indications:	• Placed contralateral to injury in protocol phases I and II for unilateral condylar fractures to limit degree of opening. • Placed bilaterally in protocol phase III.	• Placed ipsilateral to injury in protocol phases I and II for unilateral condylar fractures to traction fracture segments out to length. • Placed bilaterally in protocol phases I and II for bilateral fractures.	• Placed contralateral to injury in protocol phases I and II for unilateral condylar fractures if significant displacement is present.

Fig. 7. Placement of elastics for occlusal guidance. (*From* Kamel GN, De Ruiter BJ, Baghdasarian D, Mostafa E, Levin A, Davidson EH. Establishing a Protocol for Closed Treatment of Mandibular Condyle Fractures with Dynamic Elastic Therapy. *Plast Reconstr Surg Glob Open.* Dec 2019;7(12):e2506. with permission.)

dislocated out of the glenoid fossa and malocclusion was present. Twenty-six percent of respondents would perform ORIF with a unilateral condylar fracture-dislocation. For other unilateral fracture scenarios, closed treatment with MMF was overwhelmingly favored when the patient presented with malocclusion (90% when nondisplaced, 78% when displaced).[27]

A more recent survey indicates how treatment approaches have evolved in nearly two decades.[19] Kommers and colleagues (2015) also distributed a survey to OMFS experts who were presented with

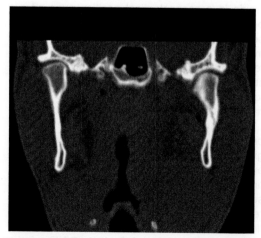

Fig. 8. CT scan image of the patient in **Fig. 6** taken nine months after MMF with elastics. Note shortening of left ramus. Patient had normal occlusion.

3 unilateral fracture cases involving each condylar level. Case 1, a displaced condylar neck fracture with medial override and normal occlusion was treated by 55.6% of respondents with MMF and 19.5% with ORIF if the patient had normal occlusion. If the same patient presented with malocclusion, the recommended treatment selected changed: 49.3% opted for MMF and 46.6% opted for ORIF. For the case of a subcondylar fracture with malocclusion, respondents overwhelmingly (81.3%) chose ORIF.[19,27]

Numerous systematic reviews and randomized controlled trials have been published over the last 25 years comparing outcomes between patients treated closed or open.[28–33] Initial guidelines for absolute indications included clinical presentations that are rare (middle cranial fossa dislocation of the proximal condylar segment, foreign body within the TMJ for example).[34] The challenge for surgeons is to stratify patients into groups based on imaging and clinical presentation that represent severe, moderate, and mild/stable injuries. Current data have helped to identify the group of patients in whom closed treatment will most likely result in good outcomes: patients with fractures lacking displacement (or minimally displaced) without ramus shortening, lacking dislocation, and/or with normal occlusion.[13,29,35] Many still recommend closed treatment for condylar head fractures but even that trend is changing.[11,13]

Indications with strong evidence supporting ORIF include the inability to establish normal occlusion during placement of MMF, bilateral condylar fractures, severe condylar displacement (fragment angulation >45°) condylar fracture in edentulous patients, ramus height shortening greater than 2 mm, and associated midfacial fractures.[13,30,32,36] It is the group of patients with more moderate presentations (mild to moderate displacement, minimal overlap but some malocclusion) where surgeons must review the literature, consult expert opinion, assess their own experience, and factor in patient wishes to arrive at a final treatment plan.

The mandibular condyle is a major mandibular growth center with significant potential for remodeling during childhood. The pediatric condylar process that is short with thin cortical bone transforms into the adult form that is longer with a thicker cortex.[37]

The condylar head in children is highly vascular and covered with periosteum with high osteogenic ability leading to an increased risk of TMJ ankylosis as a fracture complication.[3] Conservative treatment and MMF are the most frequently reported management options. The duration of MMF is shorter in younger children than in older children or adults, given concerns about TMJ ankylosis.[3] There is near-universal consensus that in young children (aged less than 7–8 years), open reduction and internal fixation is not indicated, given the risks to mandibular growth and the excellent reported results with closed treatment.[3,38] Long-term follow-up of a pediatric patient is required to monitor for the development of malocclusion, growth disturbance of TMJ derangements.

CLOSED TREATMENT

Descriptions of closed treatment methods, duration of treatment, and specific outcome measures reported vary considerably in the literature. Non-displaced fractures of the condyle with stable occlusion are well suited for conservative management. Soft diet is typically maintained for 1 to 2 months.[39] These patients undergo close outpatient follow-up to assess occlusion and mandibular function over the course of treatment.

Condylar fractures with mild displacement resulting in malocclusion can be managed with MMF followed by a period of soft diet and rehabilitation.[29,35,40] The use of arch bars is considered the gold standard of MMF, although Ernst ligatures, and intermaxillary fixation screws are also used.[40] Some protocols recommend a period of rigid MMF and complete jaw immobilization to minimize pain, provide a period of "rest" for the muscles, and allow union between the bone fragments. Duration of MMF varies from 5 to 49 days, with an average of 3 weeks reported in a recent systematic review after which patients may transition to elastics.[41]

Some protocols recommend immediate placement of elastics, skipping any period of rigid MMF, and using elastics for occlusal guidance (**Fig. 9**).[7,13,26] The stated advantage of this approach is early active mobilization which can prevent joint scarring.[7,13,26,40] On the fractured side, elastics are placed in a class II orientation (eg, mandibular first premolar to maxillary canine) exerting an anterosuperior force on the mandible (see **Fig. 7**).[13,26,40] Class I elastics may be placed on the contralateral side to close the posterior open bite.[23,40] Elastics are lightened from heavy to medium to light over 4 to 6 weeks, although they may be worn up to 3 months in some situations (see **Fig. 9**).[13,26,40]

Skeletal, occlusal, and neuromuscular adaptations contribute to restoration of occlusion and TMJ function when closed treatment of condylar fractures in both children and adults is used.[12] Dental adaptations with closed treatment result in intrusion, or apical displacement of the molars into alveolar bone on the fractured side to help compensate for this. Closed treatment also frequently results in reestablishing articulation further down the articular eminence.[23,42]

A course of physiotherapy including exercises to prevent the negative impact of scar tissue formation, to restore muscle strength, and prevent the development of chronic pain has a significant role to play in full recovery.[13,26] Active exercises require the patient to use his or her fingers to open the jaw. Passive motion exercises can be performed by stacking tongue depressors placed between the molar teeth and used to hold the jaw open maximally, progressing at intervals by adding additional tongue blades to the stack to promote adequate maximum interincisal opening

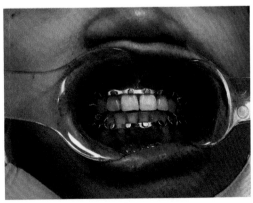

Fig. 9. Improved occlusion in the patient from **Fig. 5** after 3 weeks of MMF with elastic/occlusal guidance.

Table 1
Open approaches to the condylar process

Approach	Fracture Type	Advantages	Disadvantages
Retroauricular	Condylar head[44]	Best cosmetic outcome (scar hidden in the postauricular crease)[44] Good posterior and lateral joint exposure[44]	Risk of stenosis of external auditory canal[44] Infection can lead to necrosis of ear cartilage[44] Not advised if a patient requires wearing glasses in immediate postoperative period[44] Time-consuming, meticulous closure[44]
Preauricular	Condylar head[18]	Useful for high, anteromedially displaced fractures[18] Provides access to the most superior portion of joint and joint capsule[18] Can have an excellent cosmetic outcome with intra-auricular approach (scar hidden behind tragus)[39]	Risk of injury to facial nerve[39] Osteosynthesis plate placement is difficult because of minimal ramus exposure[18,48] risk to auriculotemporal nerve[18] No access to mandible for inferior distraction[18,48]
Retromandibular (transparotid or retroparotid)	Condylar head[18] Condylar neck[18] Subcondylar[18]	Short distance between incision and fracture site[18] Greatest exposure of approaches (transparotid greater than retroparotid)[18,48] No need for transfacial trocar for hardware placement[18,48] Scar relatively inconspicuous[18] Greater access compared to preauricular approach[39,48]	Risk of injury to facial nerve[39,44] Risk of sialocele or salivary fistula formation[39,44]
Rhytidectomy	Condylar head[18] Condylar neck[18] Subcondylar[18]	Same advantages as retromandibular approach but with improved cosmesis[48]	Longer time required for meticulous closure[48] Often requires closed suction drain postoperatively[18]
Endoscopically assisted intraoral	Condylar neck[7] Subcondylar[18]	Avoidance of facial scar[18,44,48] Lowest risk of facial nerve injury[18,44,48]	Steep learning curve[18] More time-consuming[18] Poor posterior ramus visibility[18,48] Need for transfacial incision for application of fixation[18,39,48]
Intraoral (without endoscopic assistance)	Low subcondylar[18]	Avoidance of facial scar[18,44,48] Lowest risk of facial nerve injury[18,44,48]	Poor visualization of medially displaced condyle fractures[44,48]

(continued on next page)

Table 1
(continued)

Approach	Fracture Type	Advantages	Disadvantages
		Best when used with angled instruments[18]	Difficult to determine the adequacy of reduction and fixation[18]
Transmasseteric anteroparotid approach	Subcondylar fractures[18]	Quick and direct access to fracture site[18] Excellent exposure[18] Ability to distract ramus easily due to access to gonial angle[18]	Risk of facial nerve injury[18] Poor cosmetic outcome[18]

(MIO).[43] Commercially available devices are also available for passive motion exercises. Jaw movement goals include an MIO of 40 mm (at least), lateral excursions greater than 10 mm, and protrusion greater than 12 mm.[44]

OPEN REDUCTION AND INTERNAL FIXATION

For patients who require ORIF, proper fracture classification is essential in making this treatment recommendation and in presurgical planning (**Table 1**).[44,45]

During transcutaneous approaches to the condyle, several steps should be taken to monitor branches of the facial nerve. Diffusion of lidocaine with epinephrine used before the skin incision could result in nerve blockade if the level of injection is into deep soft tissues, causing some surgeons to inject dilute epinephrine (adrenaline) instead.[31] Long-acting paralytic agents should not be administered until the facial nerve branches are protected. Continuous electromyography monitoring and a hand-held nerve stimulator are key adjuncts to the identification of nerve branches.

Release of MMF is needed during reduction to manipulate the fracture segments. Instrumentation to help in distraction of the distal (ramus) segment include sigmoid notch retractors and Bauer retractors. It may be necessary to expose the angle of the mandible through a small stab incision so that the angle can be grasped and distracted inferiorly.[18,46] A bite block placed between the ipsilateral molar teeth can also provide the inferior distraction needed to allow the proximal segment room to assume an upright position.[7] An Allis clamp or Kocher clamp can be used to grasp a medially displaced or dislocated condylar segment.[31]

Preauricular

The preauricular approach primarily provides access to the condylar head and neck. Exposure and plating of the condylar neck and subcondylar fractures is challenging with only this access. Dissection of the zygomatic arch as performed in the bicoronal approach is similar to the key steps used in the preauricular approach to the condyle.[47] The incision is placed in the natural preauricular skin crease starting at the level helical rim but may be extended into the temporal scalp as needed.[44,47] The subcutaneous fat and superficial temporoparietal fascia are incised and dissection taken down to the superficial layer of the deep temporal fascia, which is incised down to the root of the zygomatic arch. These maneuvers protect the temporal branch of the facial nerve. Subperiosteal elevation of the arch continues inferiorly to the joint capsule, which is opened to expose the condylar head. Further inferior dissection provides exposure of the condylar neck. Long-acting resorbable sutures are used to repair the joint capsule.

Retromandibular

The retromandibular approach requires dissection either through the parotid gland (transparotid) or posterior to it (retroparotid). The retromandibular vein may be encountered during this approach and should be retracted away from the field.[31,48]

The incision for the *transparotid* approach is placed a just behind the posterior border of the ramus beginning a few millimeters inferior to the lobule and extending approximately 3 cm inferiorly.[31,43,48] The incision is carried through skin and subcutaneous tissue down to the superficial musculoaponeurotic system (SMAS). The parotid fascia/capsule is opened and blunt dissection through the gland parallel to the facial nerve branches begins to reach the masseter muscle. If nerve branches are encountered, they are dissected free and retracted (**Fig. 10**). The masseter is incised followed by subperiosteal dissection of the fracture.

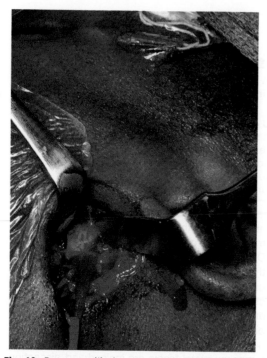

Fig. 10. Retromandibular approach to left subcondylar fracture, facial nerve branches identified.

Compared with the transparotid approach, the *retroparotid* approach uses a more posterior, extending from the mastoid tip to the angle of the mandible.[44,49] The parotid gland is encountered from an inferior approach, in the region of the tail where it overlaps the sternocleidomastoid muscle. Elevators are used to lift the gland and retract the muscles to expose the masseter muscle, at which point, dissection is identical to the transparotid route. The area of access afforded by the retroparotid approach is more limited compared to the transparotid.

Rhytidectomy/Facelift

The rhytidectomy approach is similar to the transparotid retromandibular approach after the skin incision and SMAS dissection. The preauricular incision is brought around the lobule, onto the posterior auricular skin and into the temporal hairline resulting in excellent scar camouflage.[43,50] Wider skin flap elevation, identical to that performed for rhytidectomy procedures is undertaken with broad exposure of the SMAS. Meticulous closure of the parotid capsule must be performed to prevent siaolocele or salivary fistula. The masseter muscle and SMAS are closed with resorbable suture followed by the subcutaneous layer and skin. The

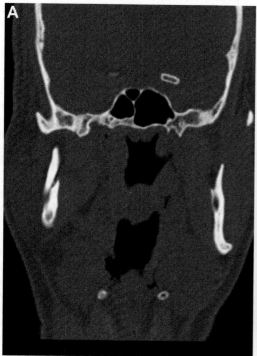
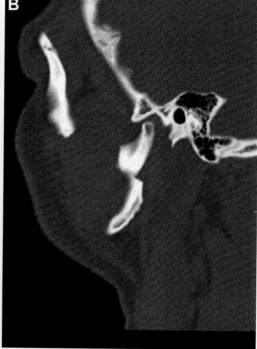

Fig. 11. Coronal (A) and sagittal (B) CT scan images of right subcondylar fracture with lateral override.

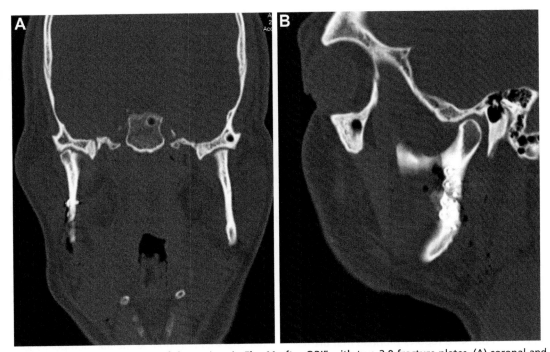

Fig. 12. Postreduction imaging of the patient in **Fig. 11** after ORIF with two 2.0 fracture plates. (A) coronal and (B) saggital post reduction images.

placement of a passive drain may be needed in some cases.

Submandibular Incision

The submandibular or Risdon incision is most often used in combination with other approaches for condylar fracture treatment to aid in distal fragment reduction.[43,44,46] Exposure and plating of the condylar neck and subcondylar fractures is challenging with only this access. The skin incision is 4 to 5 cm in length and made 2 cm below the inferior border of the mandible in a natural skin crease. The incision is made down to the platysma. Deep into the platysma, the marginal mandibular nerve runs in the fascia of the submandibular gland. The nerve can be identified and dissected free of the fascia under loupe magnification. The nerve may also be protected by ensuring a level of dissection below the submandibular fascia by identifying and ligating the anterior facial vein at the inferior border of the submandibular gland. The soft tissue flap is elevated to the lower border of the mandible and the masseter muscle is incised. Subperiosteal dissection proceeds to the level of the fracture.

Intraoral with Endoscopic Guidance

The advantages offered by the intraoral approach are the avoidance of a facial scar and protection of the facial nerve which is not encountered.[46] The addition of endoscopy resulted in significant interest in this approach in the early 2000s.[46] An incision is made along the oblique line and subperiosteal elevation is performed up to the level of the condyle. A 30° endoscope is placed within the sheath of an endoscopic elevator to allow simultaneous maintenance of the optical cavity and elevation. Once the proximal fragment has been reduced, a trocar is introduced through a transfacial stab incision at the level of the condyle to secure screws to the plate placed

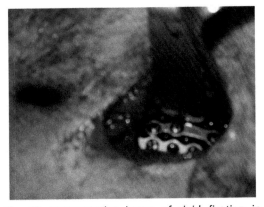

Fig. 13. Intraoperative image of rigid fixation in place-left condylar neck fracture.

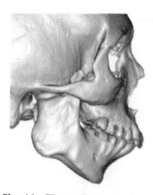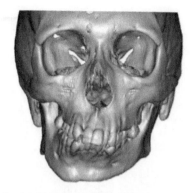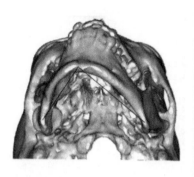

Fig. 14. CT scan imaging of a patient with missed right condylar fracture in childhood with TMJ ankylosis and right ramus growth disturbance. The red lines show the difference in length of the ramus with growth restriction on the right side.

intraorally. Mucosal closure is carried out in the standard fashion.

The introduction of angled screwdrivers and drills is an excellent alternative to the use of transfacial trocar systems for the placement of condylar fixation.[45] Published reports propose that the use of these instruments can allow transoral reduction and fixation without the need for endoscopy.

Given the tension forces and torsional forces that act on the condylar segment, stabilization at both the anterior and posterior borders of the condylar segment is recommended.[51] Clinical reports have shown plate fracture and screw extrusion with the use of a single plate.[51,52] The placement of 2 miniplates with a minimum of 2 screws on both sides of the fracture is recommended (**Figs. 11–13**).[43,51,52] This can be challenging with shorter condylar segments. For this reason, several companies have developed "geometric" 3D plates, which are designed to provide stable constructs.[51] Bicortical screw placement is also preferred for enhanced stability.

COMPLICATIONS

Visible scars from transcutaneous approaches may be bothersome to patients but preoperative counseling and preparation should help in setting appropriate expectations for the appearance. Several reviews of retromandibular transcutaneous approaches to the condyle report rates of postoperative facial nerve weakness from 4% to 27.5% of cases, with the majority of cases being transient and recovery time related to the degree of nerve injury.[30–32,49,53] If a transection injury of a branch of the facial nerve or trunk is identified intraoperatively, immediate repair should be undertaken and if suspected postoperatively, timely re-exploration may be necessary.

The treatment of malocclusion secondary to the treatment of condylar fractures is beyond the scope of this article but it is important to understand that nonsurgical, orthodontic measures may be applied to compensate for problems with intercuspation if normal dental compensations are not adequate. In the most severe occlusal disturbances, orthognathic surgery may be needed (**Fig. 14**). TMJ complications include TMJ ankylosis, joint clicking/derangement, and chronic pain, which may all require additional treatment.[43]

SUMMARY

Treatment approaches to the management of condylar fractures have evolved over the last several decades based on outcomes data showing outcomes of closed and open treatment. Fracture severity as determined by published classification systems should be used routinely in clinical practice and when reporting outcomes of research. Quality and safety measures can prevent adverse outcomes during open treatment including proper application of fixation and facial nerve monitoring.

CLINICS CARE POINTS

- Condylar fractures in children can be missed. A child with a blow to the chin and change in bite should be ruled out for a condylar fracture
- Regular (weekly) follow-up should be scheduled for patients undergoing closed treatment to monitor occlusion. Patients whose occlusion does not improve or worsens may require ORIF

- Open approaches are made safer with the use of continuous facial nerve monitoring, avoidance of paralytics, and careful superficial injection of lidocaine
- Two plate fixation (2.0 miniplate) will neutralize tension and torsional forces at the condyle to allow immediate function.

REFERENCES

1. Dahlström L, Kahnberg KE, Lindahl L. 15 years follow-up on condylar fractures. Int J Oral Maxillofac Surg 1989;18(1):18–23.
2. Smith DM, Bykowski MR, Cray JJ, et al. 215 mandible fractures in 120 children: demographics, treatment, outcomes, and early growth data. Plast Reconstr Surg 2013;131(6):1348–58.
3. Steed MB, Schadel CM. Management of pediatric and adolescent condylar fractures. Atlas Oral Maxillofac Surg Clin North Am 2017;25(1):75–83.
4. Marker P, Nielsen A, Bastian HL. Fractures of the mandibular condyle. Part 1: patterns of distribution of types and causes of fractures in 348 patients. Br J Oral Maxillofac Surg 2000;38(5):417–21.
5. Morris C, Bebeau NP, Brockhoff H, et al. Mandibular fractures: an analysis of the epidemiology and patterns of injury in 4,143 fractures. J Oral Maxillofacial Surg 2015;73(5):951.e1–12.
6. Zrounba H, Lutz JC, Zink S, et al. Epidemiology and treatment outcome of surgically treated mandibular condyle fractures. A five years retrospective study. J Craniomaxillofac Surg 2014;42(6):879–84.
7. Strohl AM, Kellman RM. Current Management of Subcondylar fractures of the mandible, including endoscopic repair. Facial Plast Surg Clin North Am 2017;25(4):577–80.
8. Lee K, Chou HJ. Facial fractures in road cyclists. Aust Dent J 2008;53(3):246–9.
9. Lindahl L. Condylar fractures of the mandible. I. Classification and relation to age, occlusion, and concomitant injuries of teeth and teeth-supporting structures, and fractures of the mandibular body. Int J Oral Surg 1977;6(1):12–21.
10. Powers DB. Classification of Mandibular Condylar Fractures. Atlas Oral Maxillofac Surg Clin North Am 2017;25(1):1–10.
11. Neff A, Cornelius C-P, Rasse M, et al. The comprehensive AOCMF classification system: condylar process fractures-level 3 tutorial. Craniomaxillofac Trauma Reconstr 2014;7(1_suppl):44–58.
12. Walker CJ, MacLeod SP. Anatomy and biomechanics of condylar fractures. Atlas Oral Maxillofac Surg Clin North Am 2017;25(1):11–6.
13. Ellis E, Perez D. 1.15 - fractures of the condylar process of the mandible. In: Dorafshar AH,

Rodriguez ED, Manson PN, editors. Facial trauma surgery. New York: Elsevier; 2020. p. 186–200.
14. McLeod NM. Towards a consensus for classification of mandibular condyle fractures. J Craniomaxillofac Surg 2021;49(4):251–5.
15. Sharif MO, Fedorowicz Z, Drews P, et al. Interventions for the treatment of fractures of the mandibular condyle. Cochrane Database Syst Rev 2010;4(4): 1–11.
16. Loukota R, Eckelt U, De Bont L, et al. Subclassification of fractures of the condylar process of the mandible. Br J Oral Maxill Surg 2005; 43(1):72–3.
17. Loukota R, Neff A, Rasse M. Nomenclature/classification of fractures of the mandibular condylar head. Br J Oral Maxill Surg 2010;48(6):477–8.
18. Fonseca RJ, Barber HD, Powers MP, et al. Oral and maxillofacial trauma-E-book. St Louis, MO: Elsevier Health Sciences; 2013.
19. Kommers SC, Boffano P, Forouzanfar T. Consensus or controversy? The classification and treatment decision-making by 491 maxillofacial surgeons from around the world in three cases of a unilateral mandibular condyle fracture. J Craniomaxillofac Surg 2015;43(10):1952–60.
20. Barak M, Bahouth H, Leiser Y, et al. Airway management of the patient with maxillofacial trauma: review of the literature and suggested clinical approach. Biomed Res Int 2015;2015:724032.
21. Färkkilä EM, Peacock ZS, Tannyhill RJ, et al. Risk factors for cervical spine injury in patients with mandibular fractures. J Oral Maxillofac Surg 2019; 77(1):109–17.
22. 3rd Ellis E, Kellman RM, Vural E. Subcondylar fractures. Facial Plast Surg Clin North Am 2012;20(3): 365–82.
23. Peterson LJ. Peterson's principles of oral and maxillofacial surgery, vol. 1. New Dehli, India: PMPH-USA; 2012.
24. Naeem A, Gemal H, Reed D. Imaging in traumatic mandibular fractures. Quant Imaging Med Surg 2017;7(4):469.
25. Walker RV. Condylar fractures: nonsurgical management. J Oral Maxillofac Surg 1994;52(11): 1185–8.
26. Palmieri C, Ellis E 3rd, Throckmorton G. Mandibular motion after closed and open treatment of unilateral mandibular condylar process fractures. J Oral Maxillofac Surg 1999;57(7):764–75 [discussion 775–6].
27. Baker AW, McMahon J, Moos KF. Current consensus on the management of fractures of the mandibular condyle. A method by questionnaire. Int J Oral Maxillofac Surg 1998;27(4):258–66.
28. Berner T, Essig H, Schumann P, et al. Closed versus open treatment of mandibular condylar process fractures: a meta-analysis of retrospective and

prospective studies. J Craniomaxillofac Surg 2015; 43(8):1404–8.

29. Danda AK, Muthusekhar MR, Narayanan V, et al. Open versus closed treatment of unilateral subcondylar and condylar neck fractures: a prospective, randomized clinical study. J Oral Maxillofac Surg 2010;68(6):1238–41.

30. Kotrashetti S, Lingaraj J, Khurana V. A comparative study of closed versus open reduction and internal fixation (using retromandibular approach) in the management of subcondylar fracture. Oral Surg Oral Med Oral Pathol Oral Radiol 2013;115(4): e7–11.

31. Shi D, Patil PM, Gupta R. Facial nerve injuries associated with the retromandibular transparotid approach for reduction and fixation of mandibular condyle fractures. J Craniomaxillofac Surg 2015; 43(3):402–7.

32. Singh V, Bhagol A, Goel M, et al. Outcomes of open versus closed treatment of mandibular subcondylar fractures: a prospective randomized study. J Oral Maxillofacial Surg 2010;68(6):1304–9.

33. Worsaae N, Thorn JJ. Surgical versus nonsurgical treatment of unilateral dislocated low subcondylar fractures: a clinical study of 52 cases. J Oral Maxillofac Surg 1994;52(4):353–60 [discussion 360–1].

34. Zide MF, Kent JN. Indications for open reduction of mandibular condyle fractures. J Oral Maxillofac Surg 1983;41(2):89–98.

35. Haug RH, Assael LA. Outcomes of open versus closed treatment of mandibular subcondylar fractures. J Oral Maxillofac Surg 2001;59(4):370–5.

36. Schneider M, Erasmus F, Gerlach KL, et al. Open reduction and internal fixation versus closed treatment and mandibulomaxillary fixation of fractures of the mandibular condylar process: a randomized, prospective, multicenter study with special evaluation of fracture level. J Oral Maxillofac Surg 2008; 66(12):2537–44.

37. Ghasemzadeh A, Mundinger GS, Swanson EW, et al. Treatment of pediatric condylar fractures: a 20-year experience. Plast Reconstr Surg 2015; 136(6):1279–88.

38. McGoldrick DM, Parmar P, Williams R, et al. Management of pediatric condyle fractures. J Craniofac Surg 2019;30(7):2045–7.

39. Vincent AG, Ducic Y, Kellman R. Fractures of the mandibular condyle. Facial Plast Surg 2019;35(6): 623–6.

40. Kamel GN, De Ruiter BJ, Baghdasarian D, et al. Establishing a protocol for closed treatment of mandibular condyle fractures with dynamic elastic therapy. Plast Reconstr Surg Glob Open 2019;7(12):e2506.

41. Rozeboom AVJ, Dubois L, Bos RRM, et al. Closed treatment of unilateral mandibular condyle fractures in adults: a systematic review. Int J Oral Maxillofac Surg 2017;46(4):456–64.

42. Snyder SK, Cunningham LL Jr. The biology of open versus closed treatment of condylar fractures. Atlas Oral Maxillofac Surg Clin North Am 2017;25(1): 35–46.

43. Loukota RA, Abdel-Galil K. 6 - Condylar fractures. In: Brennan PA, Schliephake H, Ghali GE, et al, editors. Maxillofacial surgery. 3rd edition. St. Louis, MO: Churchill Livingstone; 2017. p. 74–92.

44. Emam HA, Jatana CA, Ness GM. Matching surgical approach to condylar fracture type. Atlas Oral Maxillofac Surg Clin North Am 2017;25(1):55–61.

45. Kanno T, Sukegawa S, Fujioka M, et al. Transoral open reduction with rigid internal fixation for subcondylar fractures of the mandible using a small angulated screwdriver system: is endoscopic assistance necessary? J Oral Maxillofac Surg 2011;69(11):e372–84.

46. Kellman RM. Endoscopic approach to subcondylar mandible fractures. Facial Plast Surg 2004;20(03): 239–47.

47. Hoffman J. Surgical approaches to the craniofacial skeleton. In: Johnson JRC, editor. Bailey's Otolaryngology-head and neck surgery. 5th edition. Philadelphia: Lippincott, Williams and Wilkins; 2014. p. 1171–94.

48. Ellis E 3rd, Dean J. Rigid fixation of mandibular condyle fractures. Oral Surg Oral Med Oral Pathol 1993;76(1):6–15.

49. Bruneau S, Courvoisier DS, Scolozzi P. Facial nerve injury and other complications following retromandibular subparotid approach for the management of condylar fractures. J Oral Maxillofac Surg 2018; 76(4):812–8.

50. Ellis E 3rd, Simon P, Throckmorton GS. Occlusal results after open or closed treatment of fractures of the mandibular condylar process. J Oral Maxillofac Surg 2000;58(3):260–8.

51. Bischoff EL, Carmichael R, Reddy LV. Plating options for fixation of condylar neck and base fractures. Atlas Oral Maxillofac Surg Clin North Am 2017;25(1):69–73.

52. Hammer B, Schier P, Prein J. Osteosynthesis of condylar neck fractures: a review of 30 patients. Br J Oral Maxillofac Surg 1997;35(4):288–91.

53. Bhutia O, Kumar L, Jose A, et al. Evaluation of facial nerve following open reduction and internal fixation of subcondylar fracture through retromandibular transparotid approach. Br J Oral Maxillofac Surg 2014;52(3):236–40.

Mandibular Body Fractures

Sarah Mazher Kidwai, MD[a], G. Nina Lu, MD[b],*

KEYWORDS

• Mandible fracture • Mandible body • Maxillomandibular fixation

KEY POINTS

- Mandibular body fractures are often accompanied by secondary mandible fractures.
- A plain film radiograph may be sufficient for diagnosis of a mandibular body or symphysis fracture; however, a computed tomography scan allows for appreciation of 3-dimensional relationships and has become the gold standard at most institutions.
- Mandibular body fractures often require open reduction and fixation due to the physiologic forces of mastication.
- Understanding the location of the inferior alveolar nerve is critical in the surgical management of mandibular body fractures.

INTRODUCTION

In the United States, the most common causes of mandible fractures are interpersonal violence or motor violence crashes. Athletic injuries, falls, neoplasms, radiation-related necrosis, and iatrogenic injury are other causes of mandibular body fractures. Most frequently, mandible fractures occur in men in the third decade of life.[1] The incidence of facial fractures from sports has decreased over time due to improved safety measures such as helmets, safety visors, and mouth guards. Sports injuries account for anywhere between 3% and 29% of all facial injuries and between 10% and 42% of all facial fractures.[2] The most contact-heavy sports, such as football, soccer, hockey, and baseball are most frequently involved in sport-related facial injuries.[3] Most of these facial injuries are severe enough to require some form of operative intervention, with open reduction and internal fixation in 50%.[4]

Location of mandible fractures vary depending on the mechanism of injury. In large studies of urban populations, the angle was most affected (36%) followed by the body (21%–24%).[5,6] Patterns of mandible fractures depend on the mechanism of trauma and direction of inflicted force. Mandibular body, condyle, and subcondylar fractures more commonly result from falls and motor vehicle accidents causing anterior-posterior force. Angle and ramus fractures tend to occur from lateral force such as during assault. Mandibular body fractures also commonly occur in edentulous patients.[7]

DEFINITIONS

- *Mandible body:* region of the mandible from the canine line to a line coinciding to the anterior border of the masseter muscle
- *Mental foramen:* bony foramen that exists halfway between the superior and inferior borders of the mandible, inferior to the second premolar
- *Mental nerve:* terminal branch of the inferior alveolar nerve, a branch of the third division of the trigeminal nerve

ANATOMY

The mandible is a U-shaped structure that frequently fractures in multiple locations although single fracture sites may occur. Mandibular trauma

a Northwell Long Island Jewish Medical Center, Donald and Barbara Zucker School of Medicine of Hofstra/Northwell, 430 Lakeville Road, New Hyde Park, NY 11042, USA; b Division of Facial Plastic and Reconstructive Surgery, Department of Otolaryngology–Head and Neck Surgery, University of Washington, Harborview Medical Center, 325 9th Avenue, 4 West Clinic, Seattle, WA 98104, USA
* Corresponding author.
E-mail address: ninalu@uw.edu

Facial Plast Surg Clin N Am 30 (2022) 99–108
https://doi.org/10.1016/j.fsc.2021.08.008
1064-7406/22/Published by Elsevier Inc.

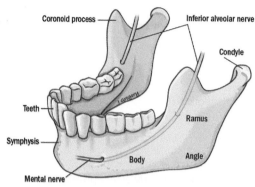

Fig. 1. Depiction of normal mandible with labeled portions—condyle, coronoid process, ramus, angle, body, symphysis, inferior alveolar nerve, and mental nerve. (*Courtesy of* Jill Gregory, MFA, CMI, New York, New York.)

often accompanies other facial fractures or closed-head injuries. The mandible consists of the condyle, coronoid process, ramus, angle, body, and symphysis, as shown in **Fig. 1**. In this article, the authors focus on fractures of the mandibular body. The body of the mandible encompasses bone from the canine or incisive fossa to the angle of the mandible and contains the molars and premolars.

The mandibular body also contains the inferior alveolar nerve (IAN), a branch of the third division of the trigeminal nerve (V3). The IAN enters via the mandibular foramen on the lingual surface of the ramus and travels inferiorly and anteriorly within the bone, exiting via the mental foramen. The mental foramen is located at the level or just anterior to the second premolar (**Fig. 2**). Just before exiting the mental foramen, the nerve will

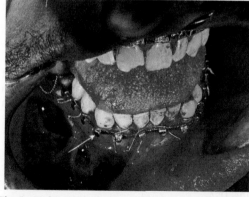

Fig. 2. Right gingivobuccal incision made to expose a right mjandibular body fracture. The mental nerve can be identified (*white arrow*) with multiple branches emerging from the mental foramen.

ascend superiorly. Thus, the level of the IAN as it runs through the mandibular body is inferior to the level of the mental foramen (**Fig. 3**). The mental nerve divides into several branches innervating the chin, lower lip, and gingiva as it exists the mental foramen. In edentulous patients, the IAN position may shift superiorly as the dentoalveolar bone degenerates.

EVALUATION

Initial evaluation of all trauma patients should be according to Advanced Trauma Life Support protocols. Airway management should be determined on a case-by-case basis. Unstable fracture segments, bilateral mandible fractures, complex midfacial fractures, and/or poor neurologic status often necessitate intubation or surgical airway. Identification and management of other associated injuries (particularly neurologic and ophthalmologic) is crucial to determining timing of surgery, as facial fracture repair is rarely urgent.

Mandibular fracture evaluation should include a comprehensive history and head and neck examination. These patients typically present with a history of facial trauma. Mechanism of injury, prior facial injuries or craniofacial surgeries, and past medical history should be assessed. The patient may report pain, swelling, malocclusion, displaced teeth, facial numbness, trismus, and/or bleeding from skin lacerations or intraoral lacerations. Lower lip anesthesia, paresthesia, or hypoesthesia may suggest injury to the inferior alveolar or mental nerve. Malocclusion is a sign of displaced mandibular or maxillary fractures, dental trauma, or temporomandibular joint disruption. As many patients do not possess perfect occlusion before injury, interviewing the patient regarding their premorbid versus postinjury occlusion and history of orthognathic treatment is critical.

Physical examination often begins with an evaluation of external and internal lacerations. Mandible body fractures involving teeth or gingiva are technically open mandible fractures. Completing a comprehensive head and neck examination helps identify additional craniofacial injuries. A complete cranial nerve examination should be performed with particular focus on lower lip and chin sensation. Gentle palpation of the mandible may identify areas of tenderness, step-offs, and bony mobility, indicating fracture instability. Maximal interincisal distance should be evaluated to assess for trismus. Normal interincisal distance varies depending on age, body habitus, and sex and is a minimum of 30 to 40 mm.[7] In the setting of mandible fracture, trismus is typically secondary to muscle spasm

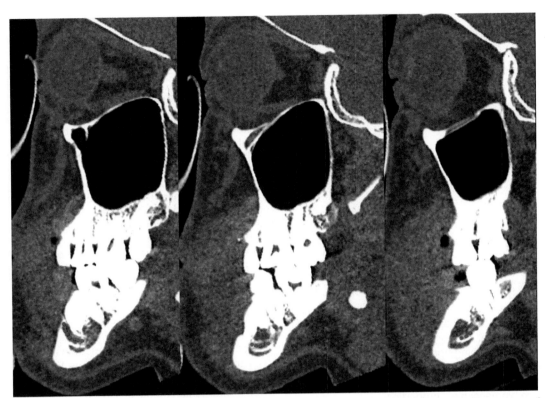

Fig. 3. Sagittal sections of a CT scan demonstrating the course of the inferior alveolar nerve. Nerve course is marked with red dots. Images series starts at the mental nerve foramen and demonstrates an inferior dip to the course of the nerve as it traverses the mandibular body.

and pain and resolves with anesthetic agents. In rare cases, a bony restriction may result in a physical block limiting transoral airway management. Bilateral mandibular body fractures can cause airway obstruction if an unstable central mandible fragment produces posterior tongue prolapse. Emergent intervention may include anterior traction on the tongue to support the airway before definitive airway management.

Preoperative occlusal evaluation should note loose or avulsed dentition. Missing dentition that are not accounted for warrant chest imaging to exclude airway foreign body. The patient is asked to bite down into their best occlusion. Originally developed for orthodontic treatment, Angle's classification is one method of describing occlusion (**Table 1**). In the setting of mandibular fractures, Angle's classification may differ from side to side and does not comprehensively describe posttraumatic occlusion. Areas of early contact or open bite should be noted and correlated with the radiographic fracture pattern. Wear facets on the teeth may offer clues to preinjury occlusion.

The gold standard for identification and evaluation of mandible fractures is a maxillofacial computed tomography (CT) with cuts at 1 mm or

less. Three-dimensional reconstruction of CT scans facilitates understanding of geometric relationships and fracture fragment orientation. However, minimally displaced or hairline fractures may be missed due to volume averaging. The axial, coronal, and sagittal cuts should be carefully evaluated for every patient. Panoramic tomography (eg, panorex) may be used for evaluation of mandible fractures and involves lower cost and radiation exposure. Some surgeons may routinely use this modality of imaging, particularly for postoperative assessment of plating (**Fig. 5**). However, the lack of 3-dimensional relationships makes appreciation of fracture angulation difficult. CT has higher sensitivity in fracture identification and decreased interpretation error.[8]

Biomechanics of Body Fractures

The mandible functions as 2 curved leavers joined in the midline with fulcrums at each condyle. During mastication, muscles of mastication apply a superior vector of force on the mandibular ramus, and occlusal loads apply inferior vectors of force at the anterior dentition (**Fig. 6**). In the body of the mandible, the masticatory forces create tension

Table 1
Angle's classification

Angle's Classification	Description
Class 1	Ideal occlusion Mesiobuccal cusp of maxillary first molar rests in buccal groove of mandibular first molar
Class 2	Mesiobuccal cusp of maxillary first molar rests *anterior* to buccal groove of mandibular first molar. Division 1: incisor overjet or labial flaring of teeth: horizontal overlap from lateral surface of lower incisor to labial surface of upper incisor, parallel to the occlusal plane when in occlusion (**Fig. 4**). Division 2: incisors are palatally flared, resulting in less overjet and more normal-appearing dental relationship anteriorly.
Class 3	Mesiobuccal cusp of maxillary first molar rests *posterior* to buccal groove of mandibular first molar.

strains along the superior alveolar bone and compressive strains along the inferior border of the mandible. Although the zone of compression favors maintaining bony contact, the zone of tension pulls the bone apart. Mandibular body fractures often necessitate operative repair due to these biomechanical properties.

Surgical management

The primary goal of management in any mandible fracture is to restore preinjury occlusion and facial appearance. For mandibular body fractures, closed treatment with maxillomandibular fixation (MMF) or open reduction and internal fixation (ORIF) is the most common method of repair. In rare cases, a compliant patient with undisturbed occlusion and nondisplaced, stable fractures may be treated with soft diet alone.

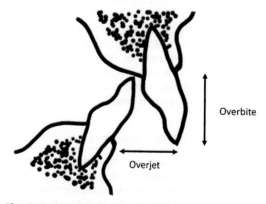

Fig. 4. Incisor overjet or labial flaring of teeth. This shows horizontal overlap from lateral surface of lower incisor to labial surface of upper incisor, parallel to the occlusal plane when in occlusion.

Closed Treatment

Closed treatment of mandibular body fractures restores occlusion via a variety of methods of MMF. The traditional method of MMF uses Erich arch bars circumdentally wired with 24- to 26-gauge wires. Interdental wiring or elastics stabilize the mandibular bone and reestablish occlusion. Heavy application of elastics may approximate rigidity achieved from interdental wiring. Hybrid arch bars are an alternative, screwed directly into maxillary and mandibular bone. Other methods of MMF include 4-point fixation with intermaxillary fixation (IMF) screws, Ivy loops, Ernst Ligatures, or Minne Ties. These forms of MMF work best in healthy dentition for short-term stabilization such as intraoperatively before ORIF. The period of MMF varies depending on age, severity of fracture, and patient compliance with soft diet. Immobilization should not exceed 6 weeks. In young healthy patients with simple fractures, immobilization may be as short as 2 weeks. Longer immobilization periods increase the risk of temporomandibular joint arthropathy and the need for physiotherapy post-immobilization to regain range of motion and rehabilitate muscles of mastication.

Closed treatment requires the patient to tolerate a period of little to no mouth opening and a liquid diet. Contraindications to closed treatment include patients with seizure disorders, alcoholism, intellectual disability, malnutrition, pregnancy, noncompliance, severe pulmonary dysfunction, and psychiatric disorders.

Open Reduction and Internal Fixation

The forces of mastication create unfavorable movement along mandibular body fractures, and ORIF is

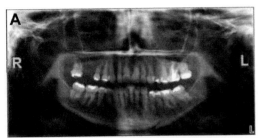

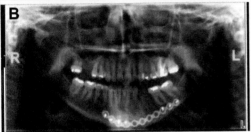

Fig. 5. (*A*) Preoperative panorex of a left mandibular body and right subcondylar fracture. (*B*) Postoperative panorex of the same patient.

typically the treatment of choice. Open treatment allows for direct visualization of fracture segments, anatomic reduction, limited interfragmentary motion, and early mobilization. ORIF may also be indicated for patients who cannot tolerate MMF.

Body fractures may be exposed via a gingivobuccal incision or a submandibular incision (ie, Risdon incision). Advantages and disadvantages of intraoral versus external approaches to the mandibular body are discussed in **Table 2**.

In an intraoral approach, a 5 to 7 mm cuff of gingiva should be maintained beyond the dentition to facilitate closure. The incision should stay just

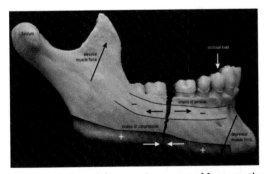

Fig. 6. Depiction of the superior vector of force on the mandibular ramus and occlusal loads that apply inferior vectors of force at the anterior dentition. (Borrowed with permission from Goodday RH. Management of fractures of the mandibular body and symphysis. Oral Maxillofac Surg Clin North Am. 2013 Nov;25(4):601-16. https://doi.org/10.1016/j.coms.2013.07.002. Epub 2013 Sep 7. PMID: 24021623.)

within the mucosa until the mental nerve branches are identified. Release of periosteum encircling the mental nerve trunk improves retraction and exposure.

In an external approach, incision is made 2 fingerwidths below the inferior border of the mandible to protect the facial nerve. Dissection should begin along the inferolateral border of the submandibular gland (SMG) capsule. The marginal mandibular branch of the facial nerve may be protected by ligation and superior retraction of the facial vein and dissection immediately on the lateral surface of the SMG. Dissection continues superiorly to the inferior border of the mandible where the periosteum is entered.

Granulation tissue within the fracture line should be thoroughly debrided to facilitate reduction. Plate selection and placement is determined by fracture stability, fracture pattern, and bone quality. For example, fractures in edentulous mandibles and patients with comminuted fractures are suited to external approaches with load-bearing plates. Alternatively, a simple, nondisplaced fracture in a dentate patient may do well with superior and inferior border miniplates.

Rigid fixation refers to stabilization of bone fragments, preventing interfragmentary motion even with active use of the mandible. Numerous options for rigid fixation of mandibular body fractures exist and include (1) single reconstruction plate (bicortical) at the inferior border of the fracture; (2) 2 monocortical miniplates, one on the superior border and one on the inferior border; and (3) single monocortical miniplate at the superior border and a heavier bicortical plate at the inferior border. In a study of 682 patients, Ellis compared the outcomes of mandibular body and symphysis fractures using 2 monocortical miniplates versus 1 stronger inferior border plate via intraoral approaches.[9] The techniques were equivalent in occlusal or osseous healing outcomes. However, he does show rare but increased rates of wound dehiscence, plate exposure, tooth-root damage, and plate removal with the 2-plate technique.

Teeth in Line of Fracture

In body fractures, there is often a tooth in line of the fracture, and in most cases these teeth are preserved. Removal of the tooth can increase infection risk,[10] and the presence of teeth helps to stabilize the fracture.[11] Tooth extraction is indicated when its presence prevents fracture reduction, the tooth root is fractured, or the tooth is completely avulsed.[12] If a tooth requires extraction, it may be used to help with guiding fracture

Table 2
Advantages and disadvantages of intraoral versus external approaches to the mandibular body

Approach	Advantage	Disadvantage
Intraoral (Gingivolabial)	No external scar. Minimal risk of facial nerve injury. Shorter surgical time for exposure.	Inferior border of mandible less directly visualized. This may result in more superior plate placement than intended, putting the IAN at risk. Stretching of mental nerve during exposure.
External (Submandibular)	Improved exposure of the inferior border of the mandibular body ensuring plate placement along the inferior border. Anatomic reduction facilitated, particularly of comminuted fractures.	Creation of external scar. Risk of injury to marginal mandibular branch of facial nerve. Longer surgical time for exposure.

reduction and achieving preinjury occlusion and removed at the conclusion of the case.

Atrophic Mandible Fractures

Mandibular atrophy occurs in edentulous patients when bony height drops to less than 2 cm. Edentulous patients are particularly prone to mandibular body fractures, as mandibular bone loss is concentrated in the dentate body and symphysis and spares the ramus and angle. In severe atrophy with bilateral mandibular body fractures, a central flail segment may result in posterior tongue prolapse and upper airway obstruction. External approaches to ORIF are typically preferred to achieve anatomic reduction and application of a load-bearing plate. Plates should extend well beyond the fracture line to allow 3+ screws on stable bone of each side. Closed treatment is possible with gunning splints or use of the patients' existing dentures. However, MMF may worsen malnutrition in an already frail population and lead to prolonged pain and impaired function.

Pediatric Fractures

Mandible fractures in children are uncommon but warrant special discussion. Most of the mandibular body fractures in children are nondisplaced due to the elasticity of the mandible and embedded tooth buds. Greenstick fractures are much more common in children and not often seen in adults. Minimally displaced fractures may be treated with close observation. Mild occlusal discrepancies may correct spontaneously as permanent teeth erupt and bone remodels with age.

If displaced fractures occur, closed reduction and immobilization is required. The length of immobilization is also much shorter compared with adults, and typically 2 to 4 weeks is adequate.[13]

The selection of immobilization depends on age and state of dental development. Arch bars and circumdental wires may only be placed on 6-year molars, the first permanent molars typically appearing at age 6 years. Gunning splint or lingual splint may be necessary if dentition is inadequate for MMF. Plate placement for ORIF depends on the presence of tooth buds, and typically 2.0 mm miniplates with monocortical screws along the inferior border is preferred.[14]

Clinical cases

Case 1 A 35-year-old man was assaulted and punched in the face. Examination was notable for jaw pain and malocclusion. CT showed evidence of a left mandibular ramus fracture and a right mandibular body fracture, as seen in **Fig. 7**. The right mandibular body fracture is not readily visible on the 3-dimensional (3D) reconstruction due to volume averaging; however, it is visible on the axial CT. Because the patient had subjective and objective malocclusion, ORIF of fractures was recommended.

In this case, 8-mm IMF screws with 24-gauge wire was used to perform intraoperative MMF with good establishment of preinjury occlusion. A right gingivobuccal incision was made, the mental nerve identified and preserved, and the fracture exposed. The bone within the fracture was debrided, and a bone reduction forceps was used to hold the fracture in reduction. Superiorly, a 1.2-mm 4-hole plate was placed even across the fracture with monocortical screws. Inferiorly, a 1.2-mm 4-hole plate was placed evenly across the fracture with bicortical screws. The left-sided ramus fracture was exposed via a retroparotid incision. This was fixated with a 2-mm plate with bicortical screws. As both fracture sites were rigidly fixated, the MMF was removed at the end of the case, and the patient was maintained on 6 weeks of soft diet.

Case 2 A 29-year-old man was in a motor vehicle accident in which the airbags did not deploy. He had forceful facial contact with the steering wheel. He presented to the emergency room with a stable airway and was hemodynamically stable. On examination, he was noted to have a large intraoral laceration of the left anterior gingivobuccal mucosa with exposed mandible and a notable step-off. A CT scan showed multiple facial fractures, including a fracture extending from the mandibular body to the ramus and a

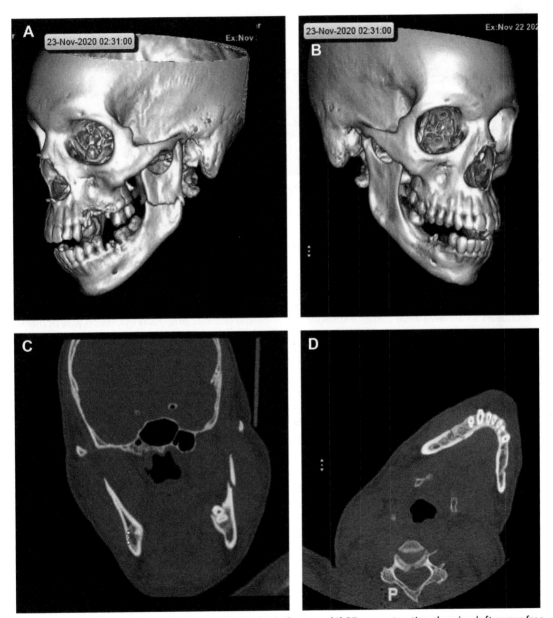

Fig. 7. Left mandibular ramus and right mandibular body fracture. (*A*) 3D reconstruction showing left ramus fracture. (*B*) 3D reconstruction with no obvious body fracture. (*C*) Coronal view of CT scan showing left ramus fracture. (*D*) Axial view of CT scan with right body fracture identified.

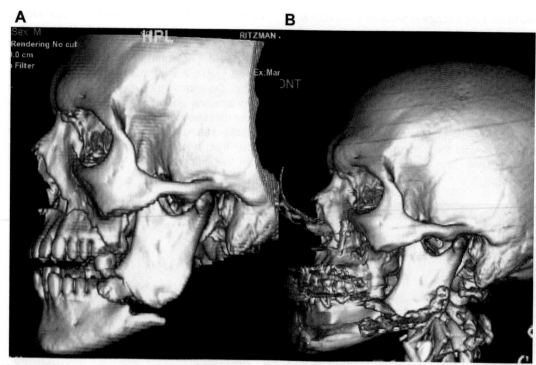

Fig. 8. (*A*) 3D reconstruction of left mandibular body and ramus fracture. (*B*) Postoperative 3D reconstruction showing reconstruction plate along inferior border.

fracture line through the second molar tooth root as shown in **Fig. 8.**

A transcervical approach to the mandible was chosen for access. Intraoperative images from a similar case are shown in **Fig. 9.** Erich arch bars were chosen to achieve MMF. After exposure of the mandibular fracture, a 6-hole 2.0-mm reconstruction plate was placed along the inferior border with 3 holes on either side of the fracture and bicortical screws. After ORIF of remaining facial fractures, occlusion was restored. The patient was kept in MMF postoperatively given commination at other fracture sites. IMF wires were kept in place for 2 weeks and guiding elastics for an additional 4 weeks.

Case 3 A 21-year-old man was assaulted at a bar and sustained a left mandibular body and right mandibular angle fracture. On examination, he was noted to have malocclusion, movement of the fracture line to gentle palpation, and significant pain. Intraoral examination showed a mobile fracture at the left mandibular body and good dentition. A CT scan confirmed left mandibular body and right mandibular angle fractures. Because of the instability of the fracture and significant pain, a 26-gauge bridle wire was placed in the emergency room to stabilize the left body

fracture (**Fig. 10**). In discussion with the patient, he strongly preferred to avoid any risk to tooth roots or nerve injury. Given his good dentition and simple fractures, MMF was a reasonable choice. Erich arch bars were placed for interdental fixation, and good occlusion was achieved intraoperatively. MMF was maintained for 6 weeks with 2 weeks of rigid fixation and 4 weeks of guiding elastics with good restoration of his occlusion. He did not require physiotherapy postoperatively.

Complications

Complications after mandibular fractures can range from 7% to 29%, with a higher risk related to increased fracture severity and comminution.[15] The most common complications are infection, hardware failure, osteomyelitis, malunion, and wound dehiscence.[16–18] These are more common in patients with diabetes, other systemic illnesses, and substance use and thus, may be less commonly seen in young, healthy individuals with athletic injuries. Several studies report a nonunion rate between 2.8% and 3.2%, which the most common site being the mandibular body.[19–21] When nonunion is encountered, the best approach is exposure of the fracture, debridement, and stabilization via fixation.

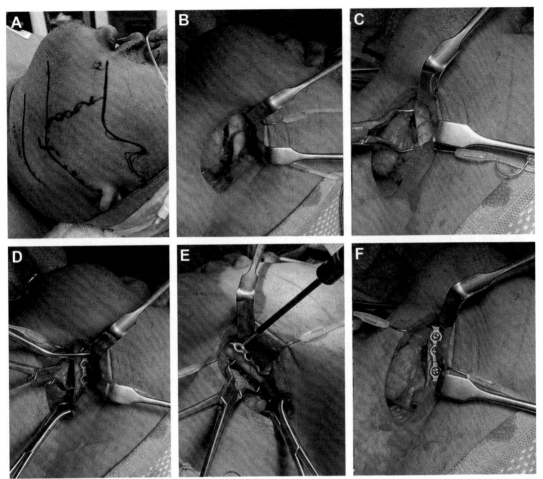

Fig. 9. Intraoperative images from open reduction and internal fixation of a left mandibular body fracture through a transcervical approach. (*A*) Preoperative markings showing mandible with location of fracture line. (*B*) Trancervical incision with exposure of mandibular body fracture at the inferior border. (*C*) Bone clamp used to hold fracture in reduction. (*D*) Placement of titanium reconstruction plate. (*E*) Placement of bicortical screws for fixation. (*F*) End result of placement of reconstruction plate at inferior border of mandible.

Return to Athletic Activity

Although there are no specific guidelines for return to play after injury, there are some guidelines that can be adhered to. In one study by Roccia and colleagues, the bone healing process was

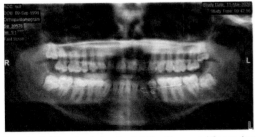

Fig. 10. Bride wire interdental fixation used for reduction of left mandibular body fracture.

noted to begin with an inflammatory reaction hematoma for 5 days, followed by formation of a callus between 4 and 40 days and a remodeling phase between 25 and 50 days. In this study, investigators recommended no activity for 20 days, light exercise between 21 and 30 days, noncontact drills between 31 and 40 days, and full contact training after 41 days.[22] Although this offers a guideline for fractures treated with closed reduction, fractures treated with ORIF undergo direct bone healing without callus formation and may be able to return to play earlier on a case-by-case basis. Slow progression of steps is ideal if the patient remains asymptomatic and continues to heal. When returning to activities with a high risk of injury to the face, protective head gear can be worn. A custom mouth guard can also be worn.

SUMMARY

Mandibular body fractures are common with multiple mechanisms of injury. They are often associated with contralateral fractures. Operative evaluation is typically preferred for mandibular body fractures given unfavorable pull of the fracture line from masticatory muscles. Thorough preoperative examination, evaluation of individual anatomy, and rigid fixation are key to success.

CLINICS CARE POINTS

- Motor vehicle accidents and interpersonal violence are the most common causes of mandibular trauma but do occur in athletes.

- High-resolution CT scans are preferred for evaluation of mandibular body fractures although panorex examination may provide sufficient information in select cases.

- The location of developing tooth buds should be considered when performing open reduction and fixation in pediatric mandible fractures.

- Edentulous mandibles are particularly prone to mandibular body fractures due to alveolar resorption of bone.

DISCLOSURE

The authors have nothing to disclose.

REFERENCES

1. Adeyemo WL, Iwegbu IO, Bello SA, et al. Management of mandibular fractures in a developing country: a review of 314 cases from two urban centers in Nigeria. World J Surg 2008;32(12):2631–5.

2. Romeo SJ, Hawley CJ, Romeo MW, et al. Facial injuries in sports: a team physician's guide to diagnosis and treatment. Phys Sports Med 2005;33(4):45–53.

3. Hwang K, You SH, Lee HS. Outcome analysis of sports-related multiple facial fractures. J Craniofac Surg 2009;20(3):825–9.

4. Elhammali N, Bremerich A, Rustemeyer J. Demographical and clinical aspects of sports-related maxillofacial and skull base fractures in hospitalized patients. Int J Oral Maxillofac Surg 2010;39(9):857–62.

5. Ogundare B, Bonnick A, Bayley N. Pattern of mandible fractures in an urban major trauma center. J Oral Maxillofac Surg 2003;61:713–8.

6. Lamphier J, Ziccardi V, Ruvo A, et al. Complications of mandibular fractures in an urban teaching center. J Oral Maxillofac Surg 2003;61:745–9.

7. Bruce RA, Ellis E 3rd. The second Chalmers J. Lyons Academy study of fractures of the edentulous mandible. J Oral Maxillofac Surg 1993;51(8):904–11.

8. Roth FS, Kokoska MS, Awward EE, et al. The identification of mandible fractures by helical computed tomography and panorex tomography. J Craniofac Surg 2005;16:394.

9. Ellis E III. A study of 2 bone plating methods for fractures of the mandibular symphysis/body. J Oral Maxillofac Surg 2011;69(7):1978–87.

10. Gerbino F, Tarello M, Fasolis M, et al. Rigid fixation with teeth in the line of mandibular fractures. Int J Oral Maxillofac Surg 1997;26:182–6.

11. Freitag V, Landau H. Healing of dentate or edentulous mandibular fractures treated with rigid or semirigid fixation plate fixation—an experimental study in dogs. J Craniomaxillofac Surg 1996;24:83–7.

12. Goodday R. Management of Fractures of the Mandibular Body and Symphysis. Oral Maxillofacial Surg Clin N Am 2013;25:601–16.

13. Amaratunga N. The relation of age to the immobilization period required for healing of mandibular fractures. J Oral Maxillofac Surg 1987;45:111–3.

14. Wolfswinkel EM, WeathersWM, Wirthlin JO, et al. Management of pediatric mandible fractures. Otolaryngol Clin North Am 2013;46(5):791–806.

15. Gutta R, Tracy K, Johnson C, et al. Outcomes of mandible fracture treatment at an academic tertiary hospital: a 5-year analysis. J Oral Maxillofac Surg 2014;72(3):550–8.

16. Iizuka T, Lindqvist C. Rigid internal fixation of fractures in the angular region of the mandible: an analysis of factors contributing to different complications. Plast Reconstr Surg 1993;91(2):265–71.

17. Anderson T, Alpert B. Experience with rigid fixation of mandibular fractures and immediate function. J Oral Maxillofac Surg 1992;50(6):555–60.

18. Iizuka T, Lindqvist C, Hallikainen D, et al. Infection after rigid internal fixation of mandibular fractures: a clinical and radiologic study. J Oral Maxillofac Surg 1991;49(6):585–93.

19. Mathog RH, Toma V, Clayman L, et al. Nonunion of the mandible: an analysis of contributing factors. J Oral Maxillofac Surg 2000;58:746–52.

20. Bochlogyros PN. Non union of fractures of the mandible. J Maxillofac Surg 1985;13:189–93.

21. Haug RH, Schwimmer A. Fibrous union of the mandible: a review of 27 patients. J Oral Maxillofac Surg 1994;52:832–9.

22. Roccia F, Diaspro A, Nasi A, et al. Management of sport-related maxillofacial injuries. J Craniofac Surg 2008;19:377.

Mandibular Angle Fractures

Gaelen Stanford-Moore, MD[a], Andrew H. Murr, MD[a,b],*

KEYWORDS

- Angle fracture • Mandible fracture • Champy technique • Strut plate • Malleable plate • 3D plate
- Load bearing • Load sharing

KEY POINTS

- For uncomplicated mandibular angle fractures, a single monocortical miniplate on the lateral border of the mandible has the lowest complication rate reported.
- Complicated, comminuted fractures or fractures that have bone loss either from atrophy or from tooth loss may require more rigid fixation or load-bearing fixation.
- Strut plates and 3D plates may resist torsional forces better, and their use is evolving as a treatment for angle fractures.

INTRODUCTION

Angle fractures are the most common fractures of the mandible. Recent reports suggest about 30% of mandible fractures occur at the angle.[1] However, the definition of the mandibular "angle" itself varies. In general, the area where the mandible body and ramus come together is referred to as the angle. The third molars arise in this area, if present, and may be involved in these fractures. Angle fractures occur in a triangular region between the anterior border of the masseter muscle and the posterosuperior insertion of the masseter muscle. The masseter and medial pterygoid muscles attach to the angle of the mandible, and a fracture can cause distraction of the bone fragments.

Presentation of the Patient

Mandibular angle fractures (MAFs) most commonly present in men and are often associated with lateral impact, such as that from a closed fist, as opposed to the anterior impact of a motor vehicle accident.[2] The force required to fracture the mandibular angle should cue providers to look for other injuries. MAF are commonly associated with facial lacerations (32%), orthopedic injuries (20%), neurologic injury (24%), thoracic and abdominal injuries (12%), and cervical spine injuries (2%–10%).[3,4]

If caused by a lateral blow to the jaw, MAFs may commonly be associated with a contralateral fracture including a fracture of the opposite body, opposite condyle, or a parasymphyseal fracture. A fracture through the angle may commonly involve a third molar tooth or tooth socket. In some instances, the third molar itself may be fractured which will have an impact on the strategy of repair.

History and Examination

Substance abuse and interpersonal violence are commonly associated with mandible angle fractures, and this type of historical information should be solicited in the history. Time and date of the fracture should be ascertained to gauge the age of the injury especially because patients who have been intoxicated may not seek care immediately. If the injury was due to a mode of transportation, this information should also be elicited, including the use of seatbelts or airbag deployment, or helmets in the case of bicycles or motorbikes. Past surgical

[a] Department of Otolaryngology–Head and Neck Surgery, University of California, San Francisco, School of Medicine, 2233 Post Street, 3rd Floor, San Francisco, CA 94115, USA; [b] Zuckerberg San Francisco General Hospital, San Francisco, CA, USA
* Corresponding author. Department of Otolaryngology–Head and Neck Surgery, University of California, San Francisco, School of Medicine, 2233 Post Street, 3rd Floor, San Francisco, CA 94115.
E-mail address: andrew.murr@ucsf.edu

Facial Plast Surg Clin N Am 30 (2022) 109–116
https://doi.org/10.1016/j.fsc.2021.08.009
1064-7406/22/Published by Elsevier Inc.

history with special attention to the status of wisdom teeth or cosmetic or functional jaw surgery is also pertinent. The patient should be queried regarding appearance, occlusion, and the presence of sensory nerve deficits.

Physical examination should focus on tenderness, swelling, lip numbness (related to injury of the inferior alveolar nerve), trismus, an intraoral step-off, and the state of the patient's current dentition. Occlusion is of paramount importance in determining treatment. Evaluating fractures in teeth-bearing regions may identify fractured dentition or may reveal lost or avulsed teeth.[5] A survey of the complete head and neck should be accomplished to be certain that fractures of other facial structures are suspected and identified.

Diagnosis (Imaging)

Once a mandible fracture is suspected based on history and physical examination, there are several diagnostic imaging modalities that can be used based on availability. Panorex plain films (orthopantomogram) in combination with a posterior-anterior plain film will provide two views of the mandible which would show an MAF, while a panorex radiograph alone may miss a posterior fracture. However, the equipment to obtain panorex views tends to be of limited availability in the hospital-based emergency room setting, and thus, a mandible series of radiographs or CT have been adopted as the gold standard. A mandible series includes three views: posteroanterior, oblique, and lateral. However, these three views may not clearly visualize the condyles. CT imaging has become the modality of choice and has been shown to have a 100% sensitivity to detect all fractures of the mandible. CT also has the advantage of assessing the involvement of tooth roots in the line of fracture, the presence of severe dental disease, and also screens for other facial fractures.[6] Additionally, CT scans can be used to produce three-dimensional reconstruction which can help with operative planning or the selection of patient-specific plating if necessary.

Treatment

The angle of the mandible has some unique properties. Fractures in this area are less surgically accessible than parasymphyseal or body fractures via a transoral approach. The cross-sectional area of the bone in this area is less than that in more anterior locations, creating less surface contact area to allow stabilization. In addition, fractures in the angle are often posterior to occluding molar teeth, and thus, slight differences in reduction can be tolerated with regard to dental occlusion. Nevertheless, the force generated by the muscles of mastication can reach 60 DN or more at the angle, and any fracture fixation technique must be strong enough to counteract this force.[7]

Antibiotics

Antibiotics given after injury, before surgical repair, have been shown to reduce the rates of infectious complications in facial fractures, including mandibular fractures.[8] However, there does not appear to be evidence in definitive support of postoperative antibiotics once the fractures are reduced.[9,10]

Conservative Treatment

Given the muscular forces on the angle of the mandible, conservative treatment with soft diet or maxillomandibular fixation is often insufficient for treatment of MAFs, even those that are nondisplaced. In addition, the benefit of early function, early mobilization, and rehabilitation is always a goal of operative approaches to mandibular fractures.

Surgical Treatment: Airway Management, Occlusion, Approaches, Surgical Technique

Airway management

Airway management in open reduction, internal fixation of MAFs is often achieved through nasotracheal intubation. This allows the airway to be stabilized without the tube restricting the surgeon's access. It also allows for the patient to be placed in maxillomandibular fixation (MMF) without issue. If there are concomitant facial fractures limiting access to a nasotracheal intubation, a submental intubation may be considered. In otolaryngology head and neck surgery practices, tracheotomy placement is a familiar technique that controls the airway without risking instrumentation of the nose in circumstances where skull base integrity is in question. Tracheotomy allows unfettered access to the oral cavity and the mandible during surgical repair of facial fractures of all types. Tracheotomy also has the advantage of being useful in the intensive care unit setting and allows for prolonged convalescence. However, a typical isolated mandible fracture without severe concomitant injury seldom requires airway control beyond nasotracheal intubation for the duration of the surgical case. One exception regarding airway control in mandible fractures may be in the circumstance of "bucket handle fractures" of the anterior mandible. This occurs when there are bilateral parasymphyseal fractures that allow collapse of the infraglossal musculature which can cause the base of tongue to relapse with subsequent airway obstruction. This constitutes an airway emergency that will require urgent airway control through intubation or tracheotomy.

Open Reduction, Internal Fixation

Single plate versus two plates

Historically, immobilization of the jaw was the gold standard of care for all mandible fractures. If a fracture was surgically opened, wires were the primary means of fixation.[11] However, the development of plating systems that allow for stabilization of the mandible with or without limited MMF has advantages. Early jaw mobility has been facilitated by internal fixation techniques with subsequent decreased concerns for weight loss, improved patient comfort, less risk of airway compromise, and faster return to active and normal function.

When approaching a MAF, several important factors must be considered. A key determination is the presence or absence of other mandibular fractures. The presence of other fractures may determine the order or technique of the approach. For instance, if there is a nondisplaced contralateral condyle fracture, this circumstance portends the need for guiding elastics, and the use of Erich arch bars will likely be the first step in fracture repair. Angle fractures are usually "retro-occlusal" in that they occur behind the articulated dentition. Therefore, if other fractures are present in the dentate segment of the mandible, it is these "occlusal" fractures that strategically are approached first. Fractures of the mandibular angle are often approached transorally through an incision proximate to the retromolar trigone or through a gingival incision that is described for third molar extraction. In the case of an isolated angle fracture, the fracture is typically completely exposed, and reduction is attempted before placing the patient into maxillomandibular fixation. Yet, maxillomandibular fixation would typically be a prerequisite to plating of the fracture as MMF is typically beneficial to achieving optimal fragment reduction. Temporary MMF techniques include the use of intermaxillary fixation (IMF) titanium screws, the use of Ivy loops, or the use of Ernst ligatures along with several other methodologies including a type of zip tie or embrasure wires. The instrumentation for the transoral approach to the angle uses transbuccal trocars for the plate and screw placement. It is beneficial to use threaded locking plates in the repair because the threaded locking plates can be secured directly to the transbuccal trocar to allow control of the plate while the repair is being secured and for drilling screw holes (**Fig. 1**). Headlights and surgical magnification using loupes or endoscopes can improve visualization during the repair.

Currently, the Champy technique for osteosynthesis is used preferentially for noncomminuted fractures of the mandibular angle. The Champy technique was popularized by Maxime Champy in the 1970s. Dr. Champy recognized that the angle of the mandible had certain characteristics that were favorable with regard to using a load-sharing engineering concept with regard to mandibular fixation. Load sharing is an engineering technique where forces caused by mandibular function will be counteracted by placing plates with monocortical screws in such a way that tensile or distractive forces are obviated while beneficial compressive forces are strategically promoted. This is in contrast to load-bearing repairs, whereby all forces at play on a functioning mandible will be overcome and neutralized by thick and rigid plates that have absolutely no mobility and use bicortical screw placement. The Champy technique uses optimal plate placement along Champy's lines using monocortical screws that counteract tensile forces that occur during mandible function while allowing compressive forces to be controlled in the pursuit of bone healing (**Fig. 2**). By using monocortical miniplates to counteract tensile forces, smaller and thinner plates can be used. Less surgical exposure and periosteum stripping is required, and less bone drilling is necessary. However, the Champy technique is not a rigid technique. It does allow some movement at the fracture site after repair. The Champy technique also relies on bone surface area contact to help stabilize the fracture, and therefore, comminuted fractures are not ideal

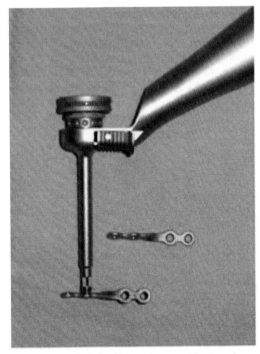

Fig. 1. Threaded locking plates with transbuccal trocar. Transbuccal trocars and threaded locking plates can be used to control plate placement during transoral access.

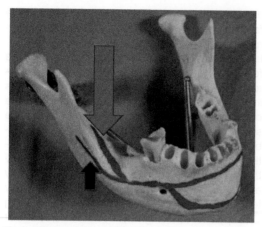

Fig. 2. Champy's lines. This mandible has drawn upon it a depiction of Champy's lines. Monocortical plates placed along these lines counteract the tensile forces at play in mandibular function. Angle fractures may be controlled with a plate on the external oblique ridge (*blue arrow*) or on the lateral border of the mandible (*black arrow*) at the angle.

for the technique[12] (**Fig. 3**). One other factor makes the angle an opportune place for utilization of this technique: the fact that angle fractures are actually behind the dentate portion of the mandible. Similar to sagittal split osteotomy surgery, the location of the angle fracture in this retro-occlusal zone allows leeway with regard to the precision of the final osteosynthesis as it relates to postoperative occlusion.

There have been numerous studies investigating the use of one versus two monocortical miniplates in open reduction and internal fixation of MAFs. Historically Michelet and colleagues,[13] and later Champy and colleagues,[14] introduced of the use

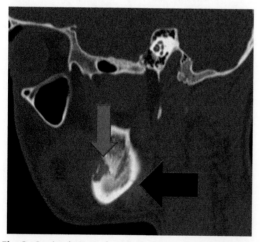

Fig. 3. Sagittal view of angle fracture through a tooth socket. The black arrow points to a nondisplaced angle fracture, and the blue arrow points to a tooth socket which decreases contact surface area.

of a single miniplate on the superior lateral border of the mandibular angle for osteosynthesis in MAFs (**Fig. 4**). However, given the tensile forces of elevation on the mandibular ramus countered by the depressor forces on the mandibular body, later studies theorized that two miniplates should be placed, one superior and one inferior across the MAF (**Fig. 5**). This has not been borne out in the literature as studies in which two points of fixation were used had higher complication rates than studies in which one miniplate was used.[15,16] A 2014 systematic review and meta-analysis by Al-Moraissi and Ellis found the use of one miniplate to be superior to the use of two, reducing postoperative complications (including dehiscence, infection, nonunion, malunion, malocclusion, and hardware failure).[17] This corroborated randomized control trials of the same topic, showing that the use of two miniplates for MAF gave no additional benefit and increased both procedure time and risk of postoperative complication.[18–20]

Malleable plates

Malleable fixation plates are a bendable and less rigid version of the classic Champy plate, have a thin profile, and similarly use monocortical screws. The plate must be bent to the contour of the mandibular arch on which it is being placed but is malleable enough to allow final contouring to be formed by the screws as they are tightened and driven home. These plates were initially intended for non-load-bearing areas, such as the mid-face, however; they were adapted for MAFs after studies found one point of fixation to be superior to two for reduction of these fractures. Potter and Ellis were among the first to report on the use of these thin malleable plates with 1.3-mm screws, and while they were found to provide sufficient reduction, there was a high rate of intraoperative failure due to plate fracture upon fixation.[21] In 2011, Esen and colleagues performed a cadaver study on sheep mandibles showing the use of a single thin malleable plate was not sufficient alone to withstand the forces generated by biting.[22] Thus, a single thin malleable plate is not considered the gold standard of treatment for fracture osteosynthesis.

Lateral border

Although not original to Champy's description, monocortical miniplate placement on the lateral boarder of the angle in a *superior* position has been shown to have the lowest complication rate in the literature (**Fig. 6**). Specifically, plate dehiscence has an odds ratio five times lower if the plate is placed on the lateral mandibular surface rather than on the external oblique ridge.[23] The success of this technique may have to do with having

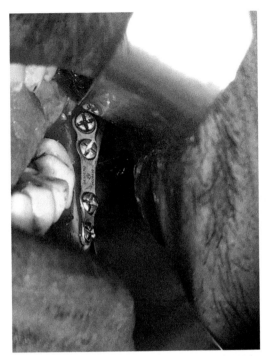

Fig. 4. Single monocortical miniplate placed upon external oblique ridge along Champy's lines. The classic placement of a single monocortical miniplate along Champy's lines. Notice that the plate must be twisted to match the contour of the retromolar trigone.

more facile operative access through the transoral approach for this position of plate placement. The Champy technique is based on obviating tensile force, and placement of a plate on the lateral boarder can accomplish that task efficiently.

The lateral *inferior* boarder also can be used for load-bearing rigid fixation using bicortical screws

and thick plates designed to bear the complete load of mandibular function. Three holes on each side of the fracture would be considered the minimum optimal engineering necessary to accomplish safe immediate function. The placement of such thick and large hardware in this position is often accomplished through an external skin incision to allow optimal exposure for plate placement and plate contouring. The choice of this technique is made when fractures are comminuted, when the mandible is edentulous and atrophic with loss of alveolar bone stock, or when there is tooth loss which reduces contact surface area. Load-bearing approaches are also preferential in circumstances where infection is present (**Fig. 7**).

Strut Plates/3D Plates, Box Plates

While the use of titanium miniplates is still considered the conventional method for internal fixation and osteosynthesis of MAF, newer techniques explore unconventional plate shapes.

Given the concerns for stability of MAFs as forces oppose each other, 3D and geometric plates were introduced in 1992 by Farmand and Dupoirieux as a way to provide stability in three dimensions. Their hypothesis was that by using an open cube or square as the smallest structural component of the titanium plate, thinner plates could be used. Thinner plates allow for more free space during the procedure, easy adaptation of the plate to the bone without distortion, and superficial screws which only penetrate the outer cortex of the mandible. Outer cortical screws have the advantage of not being as proximate to the inferior alveolar nerve while also requiring less drilling and less bone and vascular disruption.[24,25] Subsequent systematic reviews of

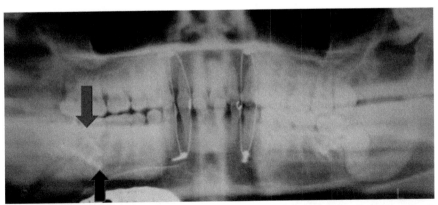

Fig. 5. Two miniplates at the angle. One plate is placed on the eternal oblique ridge (*red arrow*), and one plate is placed on the lateral superior border (*black arrow*). This is the so called two-plate approach. This technique was accomplished for bilateral angle fractures in this case. Two plates may resist twist and be a bit more rigid than one plate but have shown to have a higher complication rate. Often, when there are bilateral fractures, surgeons choose to use load-bearing repair techniques for one of the fractures. That was not done in this case.

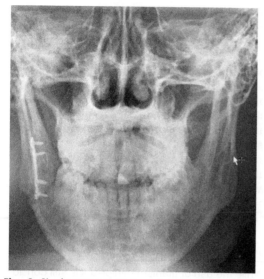

Fig. 6. Single monocortical miniplate placed on the lateral superior border. This placement of a miniplate on the lateral superior border of the mandible at the angle has the lowest complication rate for uncomplicated fractures.

this technique found noninferiority in reduction of MAFs when compared with the conventional miniplate technique.[26] A 2013 single-center study by Brisette and colleagues showed not only noninferiority but also low rates of inferior alveolar nerve injury and infection, as well as trends toward shorter operative time.[27] The advantages of 3D miniplates also include simultaneous stabilization of both superior and inferior borders of the fracture and the subsequent improved biomechanical stability.[28] Strut plates have also been shown to have a significant decrease in postoperative wound dehiscence. Three-dimensional and geometric plates may have superior ability to counteract twisting forces that are at play when the mandible is in function **Fig. 8.**

Potential Complications

In patients who undergo open reduction and internal fixation of their MAF, postoperative MMF is not necessary as long as the fixation technique is properly engineered. Both load-bearing and load-sharing techniques can produce the ability to allow the patient to have immediate masticatory function. However, if the patient is dentulous and experiences malocclusion in the days just after surgery, training elastics may be placed to guide the desired occlusion if a monocortical miniplate Champy technique is used.[8] Despite routine approach to fractures transorally, the literature does not support the regular use of postoperative antibiotics after surgery.[9,10] The use of a strut plate applied transorally is associated with a decrease in wound dehiscence in at least one reported series experience. [23,29]

Injury to the inferior alveolar nerve is a potential complication in the surgical approach to mandible fractures. This most commonly occurs when plates extend superior to the canal and the screws placed are too long. Generally, 5-6 mm screws are sufficient to engage the cortex of the bone but not extend through the cancellous bone to approximate the location of the nerve and reduce the risk of nerve injury.[8] Loosening of the embedded screws and breakdown of the gingiva over the superior aspect of the plate is relatively uncommon, although can be treated with local wound care with Peridex mouth rinse and oral antibiotics. Major complications include malunion, nonunion, severe infection, and loss of bone vitality. A 2018 study found that patients who smoked perioperatively were more likely to have a major complication, and approach to the fracture (transcervical vs transoral) was not associated with adverse outcomes.[30]

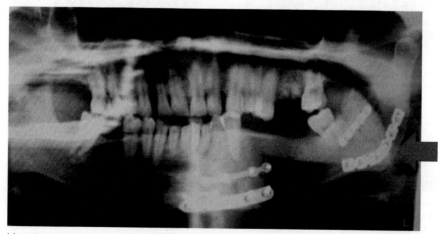

Fig. 7. Load-bearing repair. A *red arrow* points to a load-bearing repair of a left angle fracture using a 6-hole bicortical heavy plate at the lower border combined with a tension band using monocortical screws at the superior border.

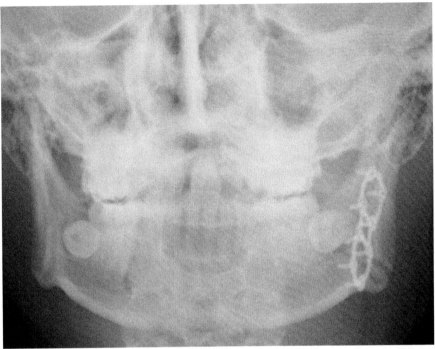

Fig. 8. Three-dimensional plate. A 3D plate using monocortical 6-mm screws adds torsional rigidity to the repair but is still load sharing.

SUMMARY

MAFs are common. They are unique in that they frequently occur posterior to the occlusal dentate line and have a smaller surface contact area than other dentate segments of the mandible. Load-sharing monocortical miniplate Champy concept techniques have been shown to have the lowest complication rate in the literature at the angle. Newer plate designs include 3D plates, strut plates, and malleable plates. The utility of these designs is still evolving but is promising. The aforementioned Champy concept techniques do, in fact, result in immediate return to function without mandatory post-operative MMF. Load-bearing lower border rigid plates using bicortical screws still have a role in treatment of comminuted or complicated fractures.

CLINICS CARE POINTS

- Patients with suspected mandible fractures should have CT imaging when available. CT imaging is important to properly engineer the repair strategy.
- Angle fractures are amenable to open reduction and internal fixation. Load sharing techniques are non-rigid and are appropriate when there is no comminution of the fracture and no loss of bone.

- Rigid load bearing techniques are indicated when there is comminution of the fracture or bone loss.
- It is reasonable to obtain post-operative imaging after fracture repair. Post-imaging serves to provide documentation of the repair in the immediate post-surgical state, provides a guide for future care, and also serves to allow the surgeon to objectively evaluate results.
- If properly engineered, mono-cortical non-rigid load sharing fixation techniques can result in the ability for the patient to have immediate post procedural function without post-operative intermaxillary fixation.

DISCLOSURE

Dr A.H. Murr is a current member of the AOCMF International Board and a past Chair of the AOCMF North American Board.

REFERENCES

1. Odono LT, Brady CM, Urata M. Mandible Fractures. In: Facial Trauma surgery. Elsevier; 2020. p. 168–85.
2. King RE, Scianna JM, Petruzzelli GJ. Mandible fracture patterns: A suburban trauma center experience. Am J Otolaryngol - Head Neck Med Surg 2004; 25(5):301–7.

3. Sinclair D, Schwartz M, Gruss J, et al. A retrospective review of the relationship between facial fractures, head injuries, and cervical spine injuries. J Emerg Med 1988;6(2):109–12.

4. Haug RH, Wible RT, Likavec MJ, et al. Cervical spine fractures and maxillofacial trauma. J Oral Maxillofac Surg 1991;49(7):725–9.

5. Morrow BT, Samson TD, Schubert W, et al. Evidence-based medicine: Mandible fractures. Plast Reconstr Surg 2014;134(6):1381–90.

6. Naeem A, Gemal H, Reed D. Imaging in traumatic mandibular fractures. Quant Imaging Med Surg 2017;7(4):469–79.

7. Murr AH. Mandibular angle fractures and noncompression plating techniques. Arch Otolaryngol - Head Neck Surg 2005;131(2):166–8.

8. Ellis E. Management of Fractures Through the Angle of the Mandible. Oral Maxillofacial Surg Clin N Am 2009;21(2):163–74.

9. Miles BA, Potter JK, Ellis E. The efficacy of postoperative antibiotic regimens in the open treatment of mandibular fractures: A prospective randomized trial. J Oral Maxillofac Surg 2006;64(4):576–82.

10. Omar Abubaker AO, Rollert MK. Postoperative antibiotic prophylaxis in mandibular fractures: A preliminary randomized, double-blind, and placebo-controlled clinical study. J Oral Maxillofac Surg 2001;59(12):1415–9.

11. Dingman RO, Natvig P. Surgery of facial fractures. Philadelphia: W.B. Saunders; 1964. p. 195.

12. Iizuka T, Lindqvist C. Rigid internal fixation of fractures in the angular region of the mandible: an analysis of factors contributing to different complications. Plast Reconstr Surg 1993;91(2):265–71. discussion 272-3.

13. Michelet FX, Deymes J, Dessus B. Osteosynthesis with miniaturized screwed plates in maxillo-facial surgery. J Maxillofac Surg 1973;1(C):79–84.

14. Champy M, Loddé JP, Schmitt R, et al. Mandibular osteosynthesis by miniature screwed plates via a buccal approach. J Maxillofac Surg 1978;6(C):14–21.

15. Ellis E, Walker L. Treatment of mandibular angle fractures using two noncompression miniplates. J Oral Maxillofac Surg 1994;52(10):1032–6.

16. Ellis E, Walker LR. Treatment of mandibular angle fractures using one noncompression miniplate. J Oral Maxillofac Surg 1996;54(7):864–71.

17. Al-Moraissi EA, Ellis E. What method for management of unilateral mandibular angle fractures has the lowest rate of postoperative complications? a systematic review and meta-analysis. J Oral Maxillofac Surg 2014;72(11):2197–211.

18. Siddiqui A, Markose G, Moos KF, et al. One miniplate versus two in the management of mandibular angle fractures: A prospective randomised study. Br J Oral Maxillofac Surg 2007;45(3):223–5.

19. Schierle HP, Schmelzeisen R, Rahn B, et al. One- or two-plate fixation of mandibular angle fractures? J Cranio-maxillo-facial Surg 1997;25(3):162–8.

20. Danda AK. Comparison of a Single Noncompression Miniplate Versus 2 Noncompression Miniplates in the Treatment of Mandibular Angle Fractures: A Prospective, Randomized Clinical Trial. J Oral Maxillofac Surg 2010;68(7):1565–7.

21. Potter J, Ellis E. Treatment of mandibular angle fractures with a malleable noncompression miniplate. J Oral Maxillofac Surg 1999;57(3):288–92.

22. Esen A, Dolanmaz D, Tüz HH. Biomechanical evaluation of malleable noncompression miniplates in mandibular angle fractures: An experimental study. Br J Oral Maxillofac Surg 2012;50(5):e65–8.

23. Laverick S, Siddappa P, Wong H, et al. Intraoral external oblique ridge compared with transbuccal lateral cortical plate fixation for the treatment of fractures of the mandibular angle: prospective randomised trial. Br J Oral Maxillofac Surg 2012;50(4):344–9.

24. Farmand M, Dupoirieux L. Intérêt des plaques tridimensionnelles en chirurgie maxillo-faciale. Rev Stomatol Chir Maxillofac 1992;93(6):353–7.

25. Farmand M. Experiences with the 3-D miniplate osteosynthesis in mandibular fractures. Fortschr Kiefer Gesichtschir 1996;41:85–7.

26. de Oliveira JCS, Moura LB, de Menezes JDS, et al. Three-dimensional strut plate for the treatment of mandibular fractures: a systematic review. Int J Oral Maxillofac Surg 2018;47(3):330–8.

27. Guy WM, Mohyuddin N, Burchhardt D, et al. Repairing angle of the mandible fractures with a strut plate. JAMA Otolaryngol - Head Neck Surg 2013;139(6):592–7.

28. Singh V, Puri P, Arya S, et al. Conventional versus 3-dimensional miniplate in management of mandibular fracture: A prospective randomized study. Otolaryngol - Head Neck Surg (United States 2012;147(3):450–5.

29. Kang DR, Zide M. The 7-hole angle plate for mandibular angle fractures. J Oral Maxillofac Surg 2013;71(2):327–34.

30. Chen CL, Zenga J, Patel R, et al. Complications and reoperations in mandibular angle fractures. JAMA Facial Plast Surg 2018;20(3):238–43.

Dental Trauma and Alveolar Fractures

Jungsuk Cho, DMD, MD[a], Alex Sachs, DMD[b], Larry L. Cunningham Jr, DDS, MD[b],*

KEYWORDS

- Dentoalveolar fracture • Avulsion • Dental trauma • Alveolar fracture • Luxation
- Maxillomandibular fixation • Risdon cable wire • Erich arch bars

KEY POINTS

- Dentoalveolar fracture can be classified into the following 4 groups: (1) crown/root fractures, (2) luxation/displacement of teeth, (3) avulsion, and (4) alveolar fractures.
- Crown/Root fractures require thorough examination and evaluation of the viability of the tooth.
- Avulsion and luxation of teeth are managed through repositioning to the original position and require nonrigid fixation (splinting) for 2 weeks.
- Alveolar fracture requires rigid fixation (Erich arch bars, Risdon cable wires) for 4 weeks.
- Special considerations must be made for the pediatric population because of primary and mixed dentition phases.

INTRODUCTION

Dentoalveolar trauma is an important public health problem that has a significant physical, economic, and psychosocial burden on the individual. It has been reported that in the United States alone, the lifetime costs of bodily injuries are approximately \$406 billion.[1] Global epidemiologic studies indicate that the annual incidence of dental trauma is approximately 4.5%.[2] The prevalence of dental injuries range from 6% to 59%,[2] which affects one-third of the pediatric population and one-fifth of adolescents/adults sustaining a traumatic dental injury in their lifetime.[2] Furthermore, studies have indicated that 48% of facial injuries involve the oral cavity, which increases morbidity and mortality.[3] Owing to the variability in accessing dental resources at various hospital centers and because most patients with dentoalveolar injuries require long-term observation and follow-up, most treatments are deferred to outpatient dental care. The discrepancy of access and affordability to indicated dental services often means that patients do not present to a dentist after dentoalveolar fracture until months after an injury and many injuries remain undiagnosed.[2] The purpose of this article is to explore clinically relevant classifications of dentoalveolar injury management and the importance of concomitant management and treatment of dentoalveolar fractures with maxillofacial fractures.

Evaluation

Initial evaluation of dentoalveolar injuries should take place within the context of a larger trauma examination. It is important to remember that intraoral evaluation is a part of the primary Advanced Trauma Life Support (ATLS) survey to ensure there are no loose debris, teeth, or massive oral hemorrhage that could lead to airway compromise.[4] Once the patient is stabilized, formal maxillofacial examination can take place including a detailed maxillofacial examination. It is crucial to irrigate and remove debris and nonviable tissue, bone, and foreign objects to prevent aspiration risks. There are several methods for examining the oral cavity; however, the most important aspect for a

[a] Temple University School of Dentistry, 3223 North Broad Street, Philadelphia, PA 19140, USA; [b] University of Pittsburgh Department of Oral and Maxillofacial Surgery, School of Dental Medicine, 3501 Terrace Street, G-32 Salk Hall, Pittsburgh, PA 15261, USA
* Corresponding author.
E-mail address: lac229@pitt.edu

Facial Plast Surg Clin N Am 30 (2022) 117–124
https://doi.org/10.1016/j.fsc.2021.08.010
1064-7406/22/© 2021 Elsevier Inc. All rights reserved.

clinician is consistency. The examination should be methodical to ensure facial lacerations, gross skeletal step-offs, involvement of cranial nerves, oropharynx, and dental examinations are appropriately documented.

It is often easiest to begin with a soft tissue examination of the oral cavity. Oral soft tissues are highly vascularized and bleed easily, thus identifying the source of bleeding is essential to help with the remainder of the examination. The soft tissues of the gingiva, palate, lips, pharynx, and floor of mouth should be evaluated for lacerations or injuries.[5] This is followed by a hard tissue examination, counting all the teeth in the mouth to ensure none was lost during the injury. In general, an adult can have up to 32 permanent teeth and children have 20 primary teeth. However, this can be complicated in children ages 6 to 12 years who are in the mixed dentition stage as the permanent dentition remains unerupted in the alveolus[6] (**Fig. 1**). If an avulsed tooth is not accounted for, a thorough review of head, neck, chest, and abdomen imaging is required to rule out aspiration, swallowing, or other displacement of the tooth.[5]

Once the teeth are accounted for, each tooth should be visually inspected for signs of trauma, including fractured enamel, missing restorations, or gross displacement.[7] After visual inspection, palpation of the dental arches should be completed specifically looking for the mobility of individual teeth or alveolar segments, which helps differentiate between dentoalveolar injury and more extensive trauma like mandibular fracture.[5] Furthermore, radiographic imaging is warranted

for the comprehensive diagnosis of dentoalveolar and maxillofacial fractures.

Imaging

There are numerous different imaging options available for the diagnosis of dentoalveolar trauma, and the choice of imaging is largely based on the modalities available and the extent of injury. In this hospital setting, trauma patients with clinical signs of facial injury will often undergo maxillofacial computed tomography (CT) scans, which can be used to diagnose dentoalveolar trauma[5] (**Fig. 2**). Maxillofacial CT allows for complete visualization of skeletal and soft tissue structures, which is useful to visualize airway patency, soft tissue infection, and differentiate between isolated dentoalveolar injury and more extensive facial fractures such as maxillary and/or mandibular fractures. However, if clinical suspicion for complex facial injury is low and there are concerns for radiation exposure, dental radiographs allow excellent visualization and have less radiation. This is particularly useful in the pediatric population where the panoramic x-ray allows visualization of unerupted teeth (see **Fig. 1**).

Periapical and bitewing imaging is useful in the diagnosis of isolated dental injury or periodontal injury.[8] They provide accurate evaluation of dental anatomy and integrity, which can facilitate dental restoring and rehabilitating. Panoramic imaging can also be useful as a screening tool for evaluation of the entire dentition in one clear image. Although both these images are clinically most accurate at a low cost and low radiation exposure,

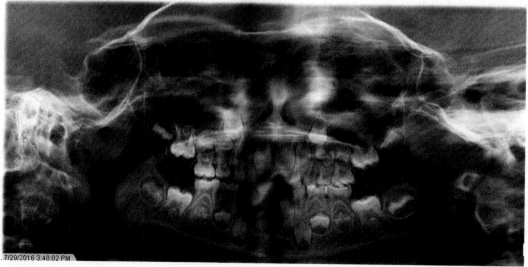

Fig. 1. Panoramic x-ray indicating mixed dentition phase with permanent dentition tooth buds in the maxillary and mandibular alveolus.

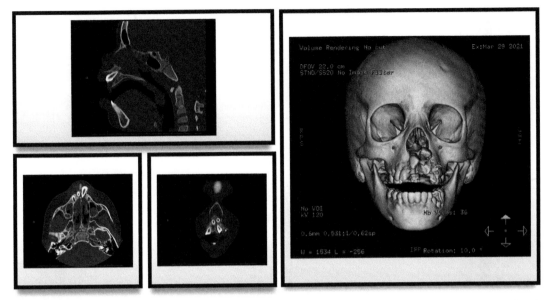

Fig. 2. Maxillofacial computed tomography (CT) indicating an intrusion of anterior maxillary teeth with alveolar fragments in sagittal, coronal, and axial views. 3D reconstruction was made using combined CT images.

they are only available in outpatient dental clinics and not the emergency room. It is important to refer these patients to dentists after discharge for further evaluation and treatment.

Lastly, photographic documentation can be very useful in cases of facial and dentoalveolar trauma. Photos allow for monitoring of soft tissue healing as well as changes in tooth coloration, which may indicate pulp necrosis and affect long-term treatment planning.[9]

The classification of dentoalveolar trauma can be classified within the following 2 broad categories:

1. dentoalveolar injury (**Fig. 3**)
2. subluxation/alveolar injury (**Fig. 4**).

Please refer to **Fig. 3** correlating to **Table 1** and **Fig. 4** correlating to **Table 2**.

DISCUSSION/THERAPEUTIC OPTIONS

The initial treatment for dental and alveolar fracture includes proper diagnosis, treatment planning, and most importantly, follow-up in order to have favorable outcomes.[10] On reviewing appropriate radiographs and performing a clinical examination, diagnosis for dentoalveolar fracture can be grouped into the following 4 categories: (1) crown/root fractures, (2) luxation/displacement of teeth, (3) avulsion, and (4) alveolar fractures.[5] Because dental injuries are closely associated with maxillofacial injuries,[11] it is important to treat dental alveolar fractures concurrently with facial fractures as

stable occlusion remains the goal of facial reconstruction.[3]

Although the prevalence of dental trauma associated with maxillofacial fracture varies depending on the literature (19%,[12] 41.8%,[13] and 47.5%[3]), it is safe to say that dentoalveolar and maxillofacial fractures occur concomitantly frequently enough that the practitioner managing facial fractures needs a working knowledge of dentoalveolar injuries. In one study, the most common cause of dental trauma was due to falls in 40% of cases, followed by road traffic crashes (33.12%), violence (21.25%), and occupational accidents in 5.63%.[10]

Crown Fracture

The most common and minor isolated injury in dentoalveolar fractures is a crown fracture ranging between 26% and 76%.[5] Depending on the extent of crown fracture which involves the enamel and dentin, with or without pulp exposure, the patient will require calcium hydroxide base and acid etch resin restoration. The extent of pulp exposure and amount of crown fracture will determine the treatment and prognosis of whether the tooth is restorable or unrestorable. If the pulp is exposed, the exposed area should be treated with an immediate temporary protective restoration and the patient will need a referral to an outside general dentist and/or endodontist to determine whether the tooth is restorable via root canal treatment or restoration of the crown. If not, the tooth may require extraction, which would require extensive

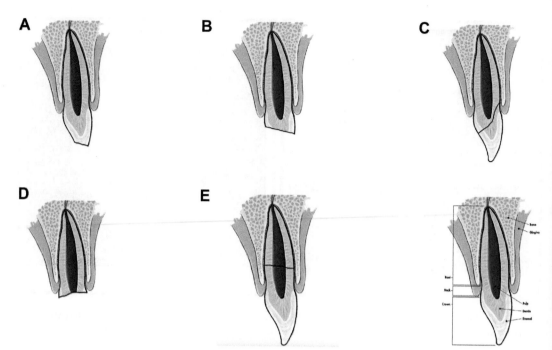

Fig. 3. Classification of dentoalveolar injury correlating to **Table 1**. (From Reynolds JS, Reynolds MT, Powers MP. Diagnosis and Management of Dentoalveolar Injuries. Fourth Edi. Elsevier Inc.; 2013. doi:10.1016/b978-1-4557-0554-2.00013-7)

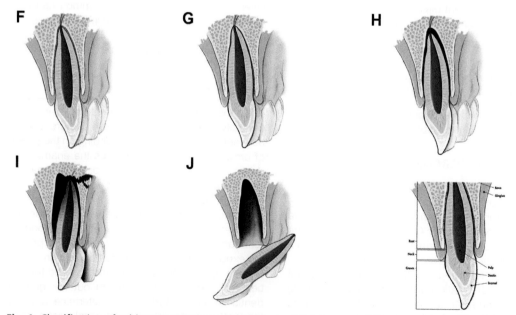

Fig. 4. Classification of subluxation/displacement (periodontal) injury correlating to **Table 2**. (From Reynolds JS, Reynolds MT, Powers MP. Diagnosis and Management of Dentoalveolar Injuries. Fourth Edi. Elsevier Inc.; 2013. doi:10.1016/b978-1-4557-0554-2.00013-7)

Table 1
Dental injuries and their definition

Type of Dental Injury	Definition
Uncomplicated crown fracture (A)	Crown fracture with loss of tooth structure involving the enamel and dentin but without pulp exposure
Complicated crown fracture (B)	Crown fracture in which the pulp is exposed, but there is no root involvement
Uncomplicated crown-root fracture (C)	Fracture extends along enamel, dentin, and cementum but does not expose the pulp
Complicated crown-root fracture (D)	Fracture extends along enamel, dentin, and cementum with exposure of the pulp
Isolated root fracture (E)	Fracture through cementum, dentin, and pulp but without crown damage

(From Reynolds JS, Reynolds MT, Powers MP. Diagnosis and Management of Dentoalveolar Injuries. Fourth Edi. Elsevier Inc.; 2013. doi:10.1016/b978-1-4557-0554-2.00013-7)

bone grafting in anticipation of placement of a dental implant requiring between 3 and 9 months for the bone graft healing alone. Ultimately, this route of restoration of oral cavity function and esthetics requires extensive follow-up and remains a financial burden that may not be feasible for all patients.

Luxation/Displacement of Teeth

The second most common dentoalveolar injuries are luxations or displacement of teeth-lateral luxation (12.50%) and subluxation (10%).[10] The luxation of the teeth is further categorized into subluxation, extrusion, and intrusion. In general, subluxation and extrusion are repositioned to their original position using digital manipulation and require some modality of semirigid fixation (splinting) for 2 weeks, whereas the involvement of a multitooth segmental fracture requires rigid fixation with Erich arch bars for 3 to 4 weeks. An exception to digital manipulation is intrusion of the traumatized tooth, which is treated most conservatively through close observation to allow for spontaneous re-eruption.[14] In the literature, spontaneous re-eruption occurs with minimal intrusion less than 3 mm; however, when there is severe displacement greater than 7 mm, surgical repositioning is recommended followed by flexible splint for 4 to 8 weeks[5] (**Fig. 5**). If the injury is severe and there is complete loss of alveolus integrity as depicted in **Fig. 2**, removal of these teeth is sometimes necessary.

Avulsion

The treatment of avulsion depends on whether the patient has deciduous or permanent dentition. The most common dental avulsion occurs in the

Table 2
Subluxation/Displacement injuries (concussion/subluxation) and their definition

Type of Subluxation/Displacement Injury	Definition
Concussion (F)	Tooth is clinically sensitive to percussion but without mobility, indicating damage to surrounding periodontal tissues
Subluxation (F)	Tooth is loose but not displaced out of the periodontal housing
Intrusive luxation (G)	Apical displacement of tooth into the alveolar bone but without fracture of the bone
Extrusive luxation (H)	Coronal displacement of tooth away from the alveolar bone, also called a partial displacement
Lateral luxation (I)	Displacement of tooth in any direction, usually involves alveolar bone fracture
Complete avulsion (J)	Exarticulation of the tooth from the alveolar housing

(From Reynolds JS, Reynolds MT, Powers MP. Diagnosis and Management of Dentoalveolar Injuries. Fourth Edi. Elsevier Inc.; 2013. doi:10.1016/b978-1-4557-0554-2.00013-7)

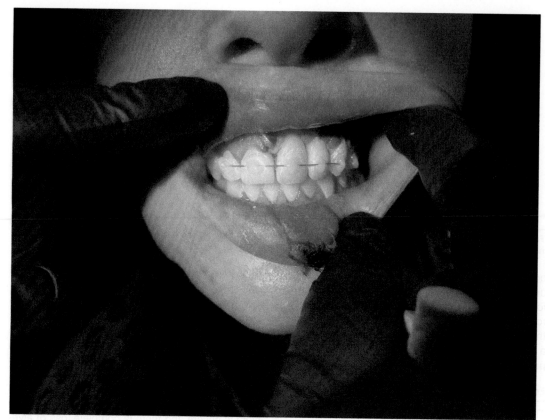

Fig. 5. Nonrigid splinting with 26 gauge wires and composite resin for luxation/avulsion fixation.

anterior maxillary and mandible teeth (49.8%). A primary tooth should not be replaced as this could lead to problems with the permanent dentition.[15] A permanent tooth, on the contrary, requires immediate reimplantation and should be splinted for 7–10 days.[5] Permanent dentition reimplantation success depends on the following: the stage of root development, the length of dry, extra alveolar storage, immediate replantation, and the wet storage period.[7] Although appropriate irrigation and removal of any foreign body material is required for appropriate diagnosis, minimal debridement is recommended around the alveolus socket because of the small tissue pedicle that provides blood supply to the traumatized area.[5]

Alveolar Fracture

Many maxillofacial traumas have concomitant dentoalveolar fractures with an incidence ranging from 19% to 47.5%.[3,12,13] If there are alveolar fractures associated with luxation and/or avulsion, proper protocols for avulsion and luxation should be followed in conjunction with anatomic reduction and repositioning of the alveolar fracture using closed or open techniques. Most alveolar fractures

can be reduced using the closed reduction with rigid fixation for 4 weeks. There are many wiring techniques for closed reduction depending on the patient's age, dentition (primary, mixed, permanent dentition), or lack of dentition. When patients have permanent dentition, Erich arch bars can be used (**Fig. 6**). Open reduction and internal fixation of alveolar fractures is indicated when an extensive alveolar fracture is associated with a unilateral Le Fort I maxillary fracture, when the dentoalveolar fracture cannot be reduced using closed methods, and/or postoperative maxillomandibular fixation is undesirable.[16]

Considerations in the pediatric patient

Pediatric patients have unique challenges in maxillofacial and dentoalveolar fractures because of concerns for growth, tooth buds, and dental variations, which makes the placement of fixation plates difficult.[17] **Fig. 1** (panorex with mixed dentition) illustrates these challenges as one can see that the primary dentition does not provide the stability to withstand the forces of Erich arch bars. Furthermore, the tooth buds prevent the placement of plates, IMF screws, or hybrid arch bars as they may damage the permanent dentition.

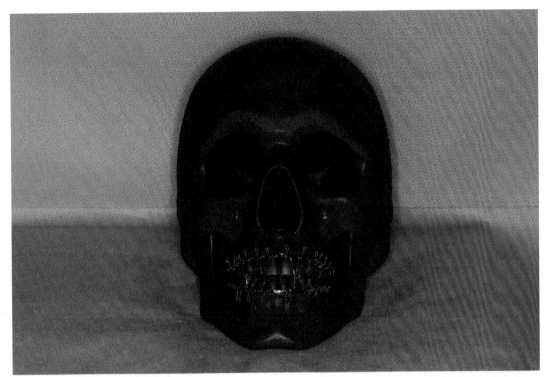

Fig. 6. Rigid fixation with Erich arch bars is indicated for alveolar fractures involved with dentoalveolar trauma. 26 gauge wires were used to secure the arch bars.

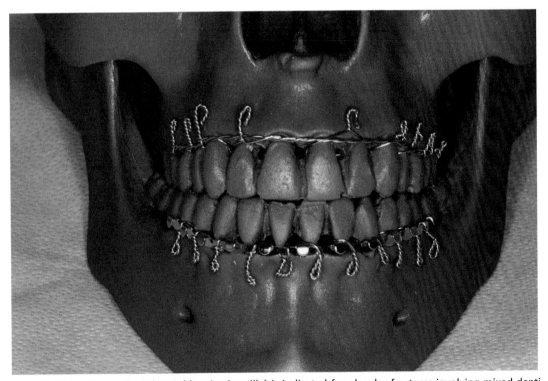

Fig. 7. Rigid fixation with Risdon Cable wire (maxilla) is indicated for alveolar fractures involving mixed dentition. The cable wire should be fixated to the permanent first molars to alleviate unnecessary tension on primary dentition.

Although nonsurgical and conservative approaches are typically recommended because of the high osteogenic growth potential and remodeling found in pediatric patients, mandible fractures with dentoalveolar fractures necessitate open reduction and internal fixation.[17] Thus, the use of Risdon cable wires (**Fig. 7**—Risdon wire) can be used because it can be easily adapted to primary teeth with fixation on the permanent molars as long as patient is older than 6 years. This allows the placement of guiding elastics or wires.[17] Ultimately, there are many techniques and variations in open reduction; however, the choice of technique depends on surgeon's experience, comfort, and availability of resources.

CLINICS CARE POINTS

- Dentoalveolar fracture can be classified into the following 4 groups: (1) crown/root fractures, (2) luxation/displacement of teeth, (3) avulsion, and (4) alveolar fractures
- Thorough examination and radiographic imaging are indicated for an accurate diagnosis to guide treatment
- Nonrigid fixation (splinting with wires and composite) is used for subluxation or avulsion of tooth for 2 weeks
- Rigid fixation (Erich arch bars, Risdon cable wires) is used for dentoalveolar trauma involving the alveolus requiring immobilization for 4 weeks
- Special considerations must be made for primary teeth and mixed dentition to avoid injuring tooth buds and arising permanent dentition

DISCLOSURE

The authors have nothing to disclose.

REFERENCES

1. Corso P, Finkelstein E, Miller T, et al. Incidence and lifetime costs of injuries in the United States. Inj Prev 2015;21(6):434–40.
2. Lam R. Epidemiology and outcomes of traumatic dental injuries: A review of the literature. Aust Dent J 2016;61:4–20.
3. Gassner R, Bösch R, Tuli T, et al. Prevalence of dental trauma in 6000 patients with facial injuries
Implications for prevention. Oral Surg Oral Med Oral Pathol Oral Radiol Endod 1999;87(1):27–33.
4. Galvagno SM, Nahmias JT, Young DA. Advanced Trauma Life Support® Update 2019: Management and Applications for Adults and Special Populations. Anesthesiol Clin 2019;37(1):13–32.
5. Reynolds JS, Reynolds MT, Powers MP. Diagnosis and Management of Dentoalveolar Injuries. Oral Maxillofac Trauma 2013;248–92.
6. Olynik CR, Gray A, Sinada GG. Dentoalveolar Trauma. Otolaryngol Clin North Am 2013;46(5):807–23.
7. Jones LC. Dental Trauma. Oral Maxillofacial Surg Clin N Am 2020;32(4):631–8.
8. Alimohammadi R. Imaging of Dentoalveolar and Jaw Trauma. Radiol Clin North Am 2018;56(1):105–24.
9. Bourguignon C, Cohenca N, Lauridsen E, et al. International Association of Dental Traumatology guidelines for the management of traumatic dental injuries: 1. Fractures and luxations. Dent Traumatol 2020;36(4):314–30.
10. Kallel I, Douki N, Amaidi S, et al. The Incidence of Complications of Dental Trauma and Associated Factors: A Retrospective Study. Int J Dent 2020;2020.
11. Lieger O, Zix J, Kruse A, et al. Dental Injuries in Association With Facial Fractures. J Oral Maxillofac Surg 2009;67(8):1680–4.
12. Hamdan MA, Rock WP. A study comparing the prevalence and distribution of traumatic dental injuries among 10–12-year-old children in an urban and in a rural area of Jordan. Int J Paediatr Dent 1995;5(4):237–41.
13. Zhou HH, Ongodia D, Liu Q, et al. Dental trauma in patients with maxillofacial fractures. Dent Traumatol 2013;29(4):285–90.
14. Reynolds JS, Reynolds MT, Powers MP. Diagnosis and Management of Dentoalveolar Injuries. In: Fonseca R, editor. Oral and Maxillofacial Surgery. 3rd edition, volume 2. St. Louis, MO: Saunders; 2017. p. 248–92.
15. Flores MT, Malmgren B, Andersson L, et al. Guidelines for the management of traumatic dental injuries. III. Primary teeth. Dent Traumatol 2007;23(4):196–202.
16. Andreasen JO, Lauridsen E. Alveolar process fractures in the permanent dentition. Part 1. Etiology and clinical characteristics. A retrospective analysis of 299 cases involving 815 teeth. Dent Traumatol 2015;31(6):442–7.
17. Madsen M, Tiwana PS, Alpert B. The Use of Risdon Cables in Pediatric Maxillofacial Trauma: A Technique Revisited. Craniomaxillofac Trauma Reconstr 2012;5(2):107–9.

Moving?

Make sure your subscription moves with you!

To notify us of your new address, find your **Clinics Account Number** (located on your mailing label above your name), and contact customer service at:

Email: journalscustomerservice-usa@elsevier.com

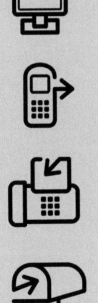

800-654-2452 (subscribers in the U.S. & Canada)
314-447-8871 (subscribers outside of the U.S. & Canada)

Fax number: 314-447-8029

**Elsevier Health Sciences Division
Subscription Customer Service
3251 Riverport Lane
Maryland Heights, MO 63043**

*To ensure uninterrupted delivery of your subscription, please notify us at least 4 weeks in advance of move.

Printed and bound by CPI Group (UK) Ltd, Croydon, CR0 4YY

08/05/2025

01864713-0014